Heletícia Scabelo Galavote

The work process of the Community Health Agent

Heletícia Scabelo Galavote

The work process of the Community Health Agent

Joys and sorrows in the space of health practices

ScienciaScripts

Imprint

Cover image: www.ingimage.com

This book is a translation from the original published under ISBN 978-3-330-74014-3.

Publisher:
Sciencia Scripts
is a trademark of
Dodo Books Indian Ocean Ltd. and OmniScriptum S.R.L publishing group

120 High Road, East Finchley, London, N2 9ED, United Kingdom
Str. Armeneasca 28/1, office 1, Chisinau MD-2012, Republic of Moldova, Europe
Printed at: see last page
ISBN: 978-620-8-03149-7

SUMMARY

ACKNOWLEDGMENTS

To God for his strength, achievements and choices.

To my father, Arlindo, who always believed in my dreams and was often the main promoter of many of them, an example of dignity, hard work and strength. To my dear mother, Ines, for her example of overcoming, joy, enthusiasm and love, and who has always supported my dreams.

To my sister, Silvia Amalia, for her support and cheering me on, and for understanding the many moments I was absent.

To my dear friend and professor Rita de Cassia, I thank you every day for the unique opportunity to meet her. She was responsible for discovering the hidden researcher in a shy nursing student, who believed that the master's degree would be a milestone for her flight in search of new horizons. For me, she is and always will be a role model who guides many of my choices.

To my dear advisor, Professor Tulio, for welcoming me with affection and allowing me to unveil theories that were previously unknown. Thank you for your patience and trust and for understanding the obstacles I encountered along the way. Thank you for everything.

To the community health agents of the Jardim Catarina ESF for their welcome, trust and the unique experiences at the heart of this work.

To all those who directly or indirectly contributed to this study.

My eternal gratitude!

1 INTRODUCTION

In other words, nothing can be a problem intellectually if it hasn't first been a problem in practical life. This means that the choice of a topic does not emerge spontaneously, just as knowledge is not spontaneous. It arises from socially conditioned interests and circumstances, the fruit of a certain insertion in reality, finding in it its reasons and objectives (Minayo, 1997, p. 90).

This study arose from the need to understand the essence of the work of the Community Health Agent (CHA), through knowledge of the ways in which pleasure/unpleasure is produced in everyday work, making it important to redefine the place occupied by the health agent in this context. The initial motivation was due to a study carried out in 2005 and 2006, the aim of which was to uncover the work process of CHAs working in the Family Health Strategy (ESF) in the municipality of Vitoria/ES. Thus, based on the experiences lived in the research scenarios, it was possible to verify the importance of a study of this magnitude that would delve deeper and bring to light the different representations of the Agent's work process, as well as the tensions and conflicts experienced in their daily work in Primary Health Care (PHC). This study revealed that CHAs position themselves in uncertain scenarios and at the same time have a large share of responsibility for organizing PHC and reorienting the health care model. There is a dichotomy between work centered on the institutional sphere and work centered on solidarity and social work, which involves working directly in the community. Through the empirical material collected, it became clear that the work generated suffering for CHWs when there was an experience of demands, limitations and violence that generated impotence and fear. On the other hand, the work generated satisfaction due to the recognition of the CHA's role by the team and the community and in relation to the concrete results that were seen in the medium and long term (GALAVOTE, 2007).

The theme of pleasure and displeasure in the workplace - the focus of this study

- is based on some perspectives of Work Psychodynamics, which is a current of thought characterized by its wealth of methodological formulations and which is built on the research of Chistophe Dejours, an occupational physician, psychoanalyst and psychiatrist, who sought to uncover the dynamics that, in work situations, led to pleasure and suffering, as well as their consequences.

The author recognizes that there is a "space of freedom" between the worker and the organization of the prescribed work itself, seen as a task, which authorizes negotiations, inventions and modulations aimed at adapting the work to the worker's needs and desires. When there is a "blockage" in this human-organization relationship, the dominance of suffering and the struggle against suffering arises (DEJOURS, 1994, p.15).

The main objective of Work Psychodynamics is to analyze the individual and collective mediation strategies employed in the search for psychic health, taking into account the subjectivity of the worker and the psychic, social and objective dimensions of the context of the production of goods and services. Dejours points out that, most of the time, the worker can't change anything in the external world and is subjected to a work organization that doesn't match their own biological and psycho-affective rhythm. He says that the tendency towards the division of labour and its standardization compromises or even nullifies the worker's potential to rearrange the task (DEJOURS, 1992).

We also start from the assumption that every worker operates according to their intentions and desires and, from this perspective, Rolnik (2006) points out that desire is constituted in the process of producing psychosocial universes and is inscribed in relationships, in which there is an encounter between bodies, which exercise their power to affect and be affected, attracting or repelling each other. These encounters give rise to a mixture of affections that are incorporated into the scenario of action of the subjects who have a flexible, experimental and procedural subjectivity, possessing an innate power of creation.

The study of the man-work relationship is therefore based on an understanding of the subjectivity that makes it up and which manifests itself through concrete and real effects, which can be visible or invisible, with the aim of understanding the meaning of work for the individual who carries it out.

The theoretical assumption, based on the literature, is based on the thesis that the degree of (in)compatibility between the prescribed work (task) and the real work (activity) can interfere positively or negatively in workers' experiences of pleasure-suffering. Thus, when there is a "blockage" in the relationship between man and his work, the impulsive energy does not find a means of externalization and ends up causing a feeling of displeasure and tension (DEJOURS, 1994). For the purposes of this study, the dynamics of live work in act and dead work described by Merhy (2007) are analyzed, in the sense that dead work can generate processes of capture of live work, in which the worker has autonomy and freedom to operate according to their intentions and desires, with inventiveness and creativity.

For Marx (1982), work is an eternal human need. It is the transformation of nature to satisfy man's needs and, at the same time, it modifies his own nature and develops the faculties that lie dormant in him. But when work becomes alienated, it loses its meaning as a vital, life-giving activity. On the contrary, it generates suffering. Although work has always been linked to suffering, it has acquired greater force today in the face of capitalist production processes. Studying this suffering, physical and/or psychic, often involves coming face to face with life and death processes inherent in the act of living and working in an alienated way.

In this context, the CHW, as a health worker, is inserted in scenarios full of desires, intentions, subjectivities and conflicts that position him as a "buffer" for the tensions of the clientele in meeting the countless health demands. However, to simplify the role of the health agent is, at the very least, to ignore the progress that their work has made, especially in small towns that until then had no access to any kind of health care (SILVA; RODRIGUES, 2000). They play a unique role as a "link" between the community and the health service, acting in accordance with the attitudes and values required by the work situation, carrying out health education actions aimed, above all, at promoting the population's quality of life and well-being.

He experiences tensions that arise in the relationship with the team, in the institutional space, and in the relationship with the community, in the extra-mural space in which the CHA is at the mercy of the problems faced by this community, developing his work process in scenarios of joys and sorrows constituted in the relationships that are composed and decomposed on a daily basis, and which at the same time constitute the being, because it is something internal to him. Deleuze (2002) presents the model of the body from the perspective of Spinoza, who considers it to be a potency, in the sense that we "don't even know what a body is capable of", and when this same potency body meets another body, "it happens both that the two relations compose themselves to form a more potent whole, and that one decomposes the other and destroys the cohesion of its parts". Thus, Spinoza leads us to rethink this encounter between bodies in the sense that we, as conscious beings, apprehend only the effects of these compositions and decompositions and "feel joy when a body meets our soul and composes itself with it; conversely, we feel sadness when a body or an idea threatens our own coherence" (p. 24).

Bringing this discourse to the study of joy and sadness in the work of CHAs leads us to think about and try to grasp the real effect of the relationships that are built and deconstructed by this actor in the encounter with other actors and to understand how the effects of this cohesion between the parties are manifested, in the sense of producing joy or sadness in the work scenarios and which will be decisive for the constitution of "being a Health Agent", of a professional identity that is affirmed in spaces of power and legitimacy disputes.

For the purposes of this study, we focused on evaluating the work process of the CHA, through the conceptions of the actors involved in the context of the Family Health Strategy (ESF), understanding the production of joy and sadness in the daily work of the CHA and recognizing that they are the result of the collective production of the subjects in activity, that is, they are constructed through the meetings between the actors of a team, or even in the relationship between the worker, the user and the community.

Nowadays, there seems to be a tendency to banish suffering from the world of work and disregard it as a contingent dimension of production. Giving visibility to suffering/pleasure is important as it is something of the subjective sphere, which differs according to the experiences and ways of going through life of each subject, depending on a certain meaning it takes on in time and space, as well as in the body it touches, producing something "beyond the pleasure principle". Thus, "the boundaries between suffering, non-suffering and suffering-pleasure are imprecise, vague, and overlap in indiscernible, often ineffable layers" (BRANT; GOMEZ, accessed August 14, 2008).

We recognize that Dejours' great merit, in considering the meaning and sense of suffering/pleasure as essential dimensions in understanding the health-work relationship, was to listen to the worker in order to understand what was happening to him, recognizing the worker's speech as a privileged instrument for research and intervention. In this way, we consider the CHW to be, in this research, an implicated subject who, according to Merhy (2004, p. 22), would be an "interested subject who values certain things and not others, who has certain opinions and not others, who has certain ideological conceptions and not others".

Based on the recognition of the CHW as an implicated subject and an epistemic subject, one who has a "baggage" of knowledge that is built up and shared through the practice of this professional, we understand that it is essential to study this actor in their real scenario of practice, expressed by the institutional scenario and the space of the community, which together make up the field of action of the CHW that could be characterized, according to Merhy (2004, p. 34), as the "scenario of the world of meanings" determined by the "nature of this arena". 34) as the "scenario of the world of meanings" that is crossed and sometimes shared by all the agents at work, showing "flaws" and noises determined by the "nature of the arena" that is set up, as well as the subjectivities of the agents on the scene and the disputes imposed.

The study of agents in everyday work, as proposed, reveals a place where there is a permanent invasion of worlds, with the production of strangeness, noise and failures, in a panorama full of meanings, where agreements and contracts exist, and at the same time where agents impose strangeness, breaks and lines of escape. Thus, observing daily life makes it possible to identify this world of subjectivities, meanings, aspirations and specific ways of producing work processes in the reality presented in health services (MERHY, 2003).

2 THEORETICAL BASIS

2.1 THE CONTEXTUALIZATION OF A PRACTICE: THE COMMUNITY HEALTH WORKER

The Community Health Agents Program (PACS) was created in 1991 and had as its initial model the experiments carried out in the states of Mato Grosso do Sul, Parana and Ceara, whose main objective was to reduce infant and maternal mortality. This experience was evaluated as satisfactory and implemented mainly in the states of the North and Northeast regions. With the institutionalization of PACS, a new "actor" emerged on the health scene to carry out health promotion and prevention actions: the Community Health Agent (ALEIXO, 2002).

According to Silva and Rodrigues (2000), the basis for the agents' privileged role in the system is the acceptance that most health problems can be solved by people trained in the short term to perform specific tasks. To this end, they look to the experience of colonized Africa, China and its barefoot doctors, the feldschers of Tsarist Russia and other similar experiences.

The ACS is part of the PACS and ESF teams and carries out disease prevention and health promotion activities through health education in homes and communities, in accordance with SUS guidelines, and extends access to information and social promotion and citizenship protection actions and services. It is a key element of the primary health care system, as the link between the community and the services. They are the ones who are in the homes on a daily basis, who experience specific health and social problems. They are the ones who witness human misery in its cruelest form:

abandonment during illness, lack of access to services, hunger that kills or debilitates. But he is also the one who has the privilege of getting to the data first, of seeing the changes that occur as a result of the intervention of support aimed at achieving health, whether direct or not (SILVA; RODRIGUES, 2000).

The profession of Community Health Agent, regulated by Law 10507 of 2002, is characterized by the exercise of disease prevention and health promotion activities, through individual or collective home or community support, developed in accordance with SUS guidelines and under the supervision of the local manager. The ACS must meet the following requirements to work in the profession: live in the area of the community in which they work; have successfully completed a basic qualification course for training as a Community Health Agent and; have completed elementary school. You must be responsible for a maximum of 750 people.

Levy and Matos (2004) state that the fact that the agent lives in the community is fundamental to building a relationship of trust with the residents, who feel more comfortable talking about their problems with a person who shares their reality. This makes the boundaries between the agent and the other inhabitants more porous, creating specific expectations and judgments, as well as defining very particular positions and roles.

According to a document issued by the Ministry of Health (apud SILVA; RODRIGUES, 2000), the ACS has the following duties: register the families they serve; diagnose their health and living conditions; update this data permanently for the Basic Care Information System (SIAB); map the community in which they work in as much detail as possible; identify micro-areas of risk, including seeking solutions to the problems identified with the local authorities; carry out home visits, depending on the family's health situation; act as an animator in the collective development of the community; work in the field of education, identifying children out of school; work in humanitarian and solidarity actions, in the search for alternatives to generate jobs, in situations of drought, floods, in the fight against violence, etc.

Its duties within the context of PHC are defined in Ordinance 648/2006, among them: developing actions that seek integration between the health team and the population assigned to the Basic Health Unit (BHU), identifying the characteristics and purposes of the work of monitoring individuals and social groups; working with the assignment of families on a defined geographical basis; developing educational actions aimed at health promotion and disease prevention, in accordance with the team's planning; registering all the people in their micro-area; guide families in the use of available health services; carry out health promotion, disease and illness prevention and health surveillance activities, through home visits and individual and collective actions; monitor, through home visits, all families and individuals under their responsibility according to the needs defined by the team and; fulfill the duties defined for CHAs in relation to the prevention and control of malaria and dengue.

They have a privileged role in the country's health system. Either because the health authorities make him out to be a kind of "joker", or because everyday life shows that he is the health worker who lives most closely with the social problems affecting health. The former try to demonstrate their importance to health from a perspective of political profitability; everyday life enables them to claim their place in the health system.

Silva and Dalmaso (2002, p. 75) state that "because (the agents) are people of the people, they are not only similar in their characteristics and desires, but also fill gaps, precisely because they know the needs of this population". They believe that the agents are the driving force behind the consolidation of the SUS, the organization of communities and the regionalized and hierarchical practice of care, in the structuring of health districts. Thus, to be a CHA "is to be a people, to be a community, to live the life of that community day by day (...)", and to be the link between the population's health needs and what can be done to improve their living conditions. It is the "bridge between the population and the professionals".

Nogueira and Ramos (apud SILVA; DALMASO, 2002) identify, in the work of the agent, the technological dimension and the solidarity and social dimension, which always have the potential for conflict. These dimensions possibly express the political and technical poles of the Program. The CHAs live with the permanent dilemma between the social dimension and the technical care dimension on a daily basis, and the conflict appears mainly in the dynamics of daily practice. They state that:

> On a day-to-day basis, agents are faced with social contradictions, which are "very heavy", and so they make certain choices, depending on the demands, rewards and their references. In the work of the agent, in carrying out actions and interactions, there are a series of situations for which the health sector has not yet developed systematized knowledge or adequate work and management tools, ranging from the approach to the family, contact with precarious living situations that determine health conditions, to positioning oneself in the face of social inequality and the search for citizenship. However, individual supervision tends to prioritize resolution, "not letting the problem get bigger"; the team meeting focuses on the individual case and the disease; the unit's management tends to have very little role in shaping the work of the team and the agent. [...] the agent sees himself as a health educator, organizer of access and the team's "scout" in capturing needs, identifying priorities and detecting risk cases for team intervention. The variety of conceptions and understandings about the community health agent and their role, held by the other members of the PSF team, the directors of the units, in short, the other subjects of the programs, shows the extent of the expectations they have to meet in their day-to-day work and, consequently, some concrete conditions for forming an identity (SILVA; DALMASO, 2004, p. 77-78).

The above considerations point to some challenges for the work of CHWs, systematized into six points: context, purpose, technology, teamwork, identity and professional training. The processes of recognizing the role that the agent plays in the day-to-day running of a service are embedded in a logic of "super-function", which would require the agent to do work that goes beyond the conceptual and practical tools at his disposal. This would allow us to say that the CHA is positioned in a space of indeterminacy and uncertainty in which there is no definition of competencies, This worker is always on the front line of the system without, however, often being able to meet the countless daily demands, since his arsenal of work tools is too restricted and does not match the broad panorama of representations and subjectivities inscribed in the daily life of a Family Health Unit (GALAVOTE, 2007).

Because they belong to the community in which they work, CHAs end up feeling co-responsible for all the problems affecting the health of this population, seeking to meet all the health needs that emerge in the context of each family, using a restricted arsenal of tools assigned to them by the USF and by the team's own professionals, limiting the possibilities for action and resolution.

The encounters that the agent establishes with the team in the USF are built without, however, there being real processes of mutual recognition of the roles of the different actors, with ruptures in the recognition of the work done by the other and with the other worker, recognizing it as a constitutive part of the collective work in health. In reality, what exists is an unequal social valuation of the different jobs, which leads us to inequality between the jobs done, which translates into relations of power and hierarchy between the workers in the different areas of activity. This hierarchy is linked to management, organizational structure, professional areas and different jobs, which generates relations of command and maintenance of the *status quo,* reproducing the technical-social division of the modes of production (GALAVOTE, 2007).

There is a disproportion between the profile seen as real and the profile expected, which leads the agent to make countless efforts to overcome the limitations and incompetence identified, which is one of the biggest causes of daily suffering. In a study carried out in 2007 by USP, four types of overlapping pressure were identified in the daily lives of CHAs: the assumptions of the ESF, from the perspective of comprehensiveness and responsibility for the micro-area; the team's professionals, which involves the need for interdisciplinary contractuality; the community, which demands, questions, challenges and claims its rights and; the agent himself, who circulates in "fantasy", being "numbed by omnipotence" (MARTINES; CHAVES, 2007, p. 433). 432).

In this regard, Lunardello (2004) points out that there is suffering in this duality of the work of the agent, who brings with him idealizations based on very high expectations of his competence, often disregarding the attributions of the team, other individuals and families, and becoming uncomfortable with the limitations of his work.

We believe that the CHW is an active professional in mobilizing and improving the population's ability to take care of their health and becomes an essential player in identifying the health needs of individuals. Carvalho (apud LUNARDELO, 2004), through a study of the practice of this professional, states that the CHA favors welcoming and rescues the integrality of the subject/user, with emphasis on the social support offered to the population through its solidarity profile. Thus, the production of knowledge and the practices of CHAs should provide endless possibilities for relationships with others and with oneself in order to enhance the production of health linked to citizenship, the autonomy of individuals and communities in the ways in which, on a daily basis, new ways of living and dealing with life are constructed, including in the institutional spaces where the various and differentiated models of health work are constructed.

2.2 THE HEALTH WORK PROCESS: WEBS, NETWORKS AND PLOTS

(...) within the health work process, the relationships that are established between object, instrument and product, in the face of the needs suggested and which direct its purpose, are directed by the intentionality of the work in the face of a certain operative knowledge that directs the agents towards the fulfillment of a certain project of life in society (NEMES apud MERHY, 2007, 108).

Throughout history, work has acquired different meanings. Etymologically, the word work comes from the Latin *tripalium, the* name given to a Roman instrument of torture on which slaves were beaten. In all Latin languages and even in the Anglo-Saxon language, the term has acquired the meaning of "torment, agony and suffering". Bom Sucesso (apud LIMA, 2001) states that until Christianity, work had an implicit meaning of distancing oneself from the divine order, distancing oneself from God, which was based on the idea that through work it would be possible to become rich, a privilege that was conditional on the power of the church and the nobility. The idea of work as a result of human production is found in Genesis, chapter three, as a condemnation of Adam and Eve for having fallen into temptation, disobeying divine orders. With the Protestant Reformation, a new value was added to work and its role in people's lives, being "seen as liberation from idleness, from sin, from the empty mind; thus having the pedagogical function of increasing the value of man, by creating a new ethic in which the product of work is then seen as a reward" (LIMA, 2001, p. 73). Thus, the logic of work as a vocation was introduced, which was supported by a capitalist ideology that aimed to increase production and profit.

In Marx's definition,

> The labor process is an activity oriented towards a useful end to produce use values, the appropriation of the natural to satisfy human needs, the universal condition between man and nature, the eternal natural condition of human life (MARX, 1996, p.303).

Work comes to be seen as constitutive of the human being, in the sense that man, through his work and the means and instruments he uses, acts on nature, modifying it at the same time as he modifies himself. It has the essential function of re-signifying the "way of acting and thinking in the world" (MERHY; FRANCO, 2006, p. 277).

The work process, like any method, technique or procedure that usually serves as a means to a useful end, constitutes the field of micropolitics and must be understood as a scenario of power struggles that emerge from the relationships between subjects, who are essentially desirous (MERHY, 2007). It also represents a technical, social and economic process, consisting of work instruments, the result of class relations and scientific-technological development, since the mode of production of work processes does not depend solely on technology, but is basically the historical product of the dominant social relations in these societies (COHN; MARSIGLIA, 1993). According to Merhy (2007), this space of the micropolitics of the work process does not include the idea of "impotence", since it is always open to the dynamics of living work that bring with them gains in autonomy, inventiveness and creativity on the part of the worker, who is above all eager to produce something, to produce the new.

Marx (apud BORGES; MOULIN; ARAUJO, 2001, p.15) points to work as being "a human activity carried out to produce and reproduce life, considering the material and concrete conditions available to us". According to this idea, work "in addition to providing material survival for men and women, is experienced as an ideal, a possibility of ascension, recognition and belonging to a social group". The author thinks of work as a form that belongs exclusively to man, exemplifying this through the significance of the work of the bee in comparison to that of the architect, emphasizing that although the bee does an enviable architectural job in the construction of the combs and their hives, it does so through a predetermined code, which inevitably always generates the same product, "the hive with its combs, formed by the drawings and with the same sizes and, as a general rule, produced with the same materials". On the contrary, the architect builds the "combs" in his head beforehand, thinking in advance about the product that will be made and that has already been built mentally, which determines an action based on an "interested cut-out" of the world, man being a living result of work in its potency (MERHY, 2007, p. 81).

Cohn and Marsiglia (1993) state that the advent of capitalism transformed, above all, the relationship between man and nature and between men and women, which led to the private appropriation of the means of production by part of society and the exploitation of the labor of significant segments of the population. The accumulation of capital, as a result of this process, demanded control of the work process through the division of tasks and the separation of those of conception from those of execution of the work, dispossessing the worker of his know-how and; an increase in work productivity through the development of work tools.

Merhy (2007, p. 82), when talking about the "human world of work", uses as an example the work of the craftsman carpenter and his tools or working instruments. To do this, he looks to Marxist theory for the idea of living work and dead work, in the sense that dead work would be the result of previous work, represented by the products involved, be they the raw material or the tools; in the case of the craftsman, the hammer and the wood. Living work would be that which is carried out in act, creative, inventive work, which is in action. In this context, he highlights the processes of capture that living work can undergo by the established logic of dead work, which generates a "crystallization of this living work". Taylor recognized that in this capture of living work, workers opened up "lines of escape" in production, in other words, he admitted the decapture of living work and sought management methods that would prevent workers from exercising their autonomy and freedom (MERHY, 2002).

Work itself would be seen as a producer of use or exchange values. In Marx's conception (1982, p. 26), the final object of labor would be an external object that satisfies needs, whether of the worker or the consumer. Use value is represented by utility, purpose. Exchange value appears as a quantitative relationship whereby the use values of one commodity are exchanged for the use values of another. The end product of labor, then, with a use and exchange value, represents human effort, "human labor is accumulated there". In this sense, "nothing can have value without being an object of use; if it is useless, the work contained in it is equally useless, does not count as work and generates absolutely no value".

Transposing the discussion of values to the field of health, Campos (apud MERHY, 2007) points out that the user seeks out a service in order to consume something, which in this case is health care, which has a use value that is fundamental to them as it allows them to restore or maintain their health. At the same time, in this relationship, the end product also has an exchange value if we consider that this establishes a mutual construction of affections, reciprocity and recognition, with concrete and valid effects for both the worker and the user.

According to Pires (apud BRITO, 2005), health work is:

> Work is essential to human life and is part of the service sector. It is work in the sphere of non-material production, which is completed in the act of its realization. It does not result in a material product, which is independent of the production process and can be sold on the market. The product is inseparable from the process that produces it; it is the very realization of the activity (BRITO, 2005, p.85).

It is work that operates in act, in which the product is simultaneously constructed and consumed, established through "intercessory relationships". Thus health work is essentially relational, it is constituted in the encounter between the worker and the user in the space of micropolitics, a space of disputes, desires, intentions, agreements and agency. What operates are "relationships of shared intercession", in which the user is part of the process, an agent of care (MERHY, 2002). According to Matus (apud

MERHY, 2007), this living work that operates in the act is "governed" by the different social actors, be they workers or users, each with their own tools for action and management of the daily work that is done in the act. Thus, Merhy points out that living work in action is always linked to the analysis of the practices of the subjects "in (of)" action and the set of tools that help to think about this practice.

From this point of view, the work that emerges in the field of health cannot be compared to the work that takes place in industry, since the former is not carried out on things or objects; on the contrary, it is carried out on people through a basis of interrelationship in which the consumer contributes to the process, and is part of it, building the space of the micropolitics of health work. Thus, health work cannot be globally captured by the logic of dead work, expressed in equipment and structured technological knowledge, because its object is not fully structured and its most strategic technologies of action are configured as processes of intervention in action, operating as technologies of relationships, encounters and subjectivities, beyond structured technological knowledge, involving a degree of freedom (MERHY, 2002).

Based on an understanding of the technologies used in the production of health services as "operating knowledge", Merhy clarifies that technology is not limited to machines and equipment, but also refers to the knowledge constituted to produce products and to organize production processes, as well as the inter-human dimension. He classifies the technologies involved in health work as: "soft (technologies of relationships - welcoming, bonding and autonomy), hard (structured knowledge) and hard (technological equipment - machines, norms and organizational structures)". In the production of care in the daily life of institutions, these three technologies must coexist in a balanced way, with the soft technologies occupying a central place since they produce the shared intercession that allows the worker/user encounter in meeting the different health needs that are, above all, socially constructed (MERHY, apud GONSALVES, 2005, p. 83).

There is an encounter between the producing agent and their tools (knowledge, equipment) and the user, who is also an agent with their own intentions and representations (MERHY, 2003). The author also points out that the new model of care that is so much sought after can be understood from the guidelines of welcoming, linkage and accountability with regard to the production of care and autonomy, which means having as the expected result of the production of care, "gains in user autonomy", which is the "key" element of the whole process. Thus, the encounter between the producing agent and the consuming agent promotes a continuous interaction of intentions, knowledge and representations, configuring a "state" of shared intersection, operating relations of encounter between subjectivities.

The space of shared intersection, as described by Merhy, is the place that highlights the instituting forces, such as needs, and the way in which, socially, the instituted process captures or annuls these distinct forces. In the field of health, the space of intersection will always be shared by the agents in action, who generate noise within it. Thus, it will be formed as a space of voices, listenings, silences and the meeting place between two constituents: the user and the health worker, who want to speak and be heard according to their needs (MERHY, 2004; LIMA, 2001).

From this perspective, Peduzzi points out that "health work is configured as reflective work, aimed at preventing, maintaining or restoring something essential to society as a whole". As reflexive work, it is full of uncertainties and therefore cannot be totally defined a priori, nor can it be subjected to inflexible production criteria (PEDUZZI, 1998, p. 83). He also defends the position that it is necessary to think about and propose ways of organizing work that have an impact on the quality of care and, at the same time, consider the possibility of carrying out interdisciplinary work that is creative and integrates the wealth of diversity in the training of health professionals.

Merhy (2003) states that the organization of work in multi-professional teams is justified in two ways: breaking the common routine of dividing up health work according to vertical cuts and; making each of these teams responsible for a set of well-defined problems and capable of solving them, which would occur through the creation of a link between each team and a certain number of users. Franco (2006) states that "establishing relationships is an intrinsic part of work" in the sense that there is no such thing as "self-sufficiency in health work, i.e. no worker can say that they alone can achieve a satisfactory level of resolution", which requires the constitution of care in a network, which allows the sharing of different nuclei of knowledge and singular potentials in order to achieve a final product that is the result of the encounters that take place in the day-to-day running of the services: care.

Another central issue, according to Merhy and Franco (apud CREVELIM, 2005), is the fact that until workers interact with each other, exchanging knowledge and articulating a "field of care production" that is common to the majority of workers, teamwork cannot be said to exist. Trapping everyone in their own "specific core" of knowledge and practices traps the work process in the rigid structures of structured technical knowledge, making it dependent dead work. On the contrary, the "field of competence" or "field of care", in addition to interaction, opens up the possibility for everyone to use all their creative potential in their relationship with the user, so that together they can produce care. This makes it necessary to produce new groups of workers who are ethically and politically committed to the radical defense of individual and collective life.

Franco (2006, p. 1) confirms that the hegemony of living work in the field of micropolitics reveals "an extremely rich, dynamic, creative, unstructured and highly inventive world". He points out that health work is eminently work that is produced in networks, connections and flows and that it resembles a Rhizome, a concept from Botany appropriated by Deleuze and Guattari, which represents open systems of connections that move through social spaces through various agencies. Thus,

> Living work, as a device for the formation of connective flows, maps the interior of work processes like a drawing of an open map, with multiple connections, which transit through different territories, takes on characteristics of multiplicity and heterogeneity, and is capable of operating with a high degree of creativity (FRANCO, 2006, p. 2).

These constitutive networks of living work in act, which operate through the connections they establish with each other, build the lines of production of care that are externalized in multiple directions (FRANCO, 2006). Considering that care is the final essence of all acts in health and that it is produced in networks, Teixeira (apud BARROS, 2008, p. 284) states that in all acts of care there are always negotiations and agreements between the "prescriptions of the agencies and the norms of the singular subjects, which are redefined all the time". He proposes thinking about care based on an idea of a Clinic that is built on a radical restructuring of hegemonic biomedical rationality. It is a Clinic based on the relationship of recognition with the other, who is not transformed into an object, but who positions himself as an actor who governs the care produced, in an effort to overcome the "I-other split". Barros (2008) seeks to relate an idea of the individual as an action, a process, a product, who has a subjectivity that makes them unique in the field of care production. He also warns, based on a text by Baptista (1999), that we need to know how to identify "who are the knife sharpeners?". Baptista tells us that these sharpeners are often invisible in everyday life and that they coexist with us on a daily basis. They act complacently, microscopically and carefully, defending a humanism that has an image of man as weak, apathetic, powerless, ineffectual, perplexed and in need of permanent tutelage. They "sharpen the knife and weaken the victim", denying their role in the construction of care, taking away from life the experience of experimentation and collective creation. These knife sharpeners deprive individuals of their knowledge-power, stripping living of its character as a political struggle and the affirmation of unique ways of existing.

Barros (2008, p. 285) states that the act of caring requires a continuous openness to the exercise of alterity, of collective construction, therefore, "as a work-in-progress, always open to new compositions where the plasticity of life becomes an ally in the invention of new ways of existing". He concludes with the observation that "it is not possible to think about changes in the ways of caring if we don't radically change the way we work in health, if we don't refuse to be knife sharpeners" (p. 291).

The professional-centered work process, tied to the specific competencies of each one of them and restricted to the production of procedures, practically eliminates the caring dimension. The challenge of changing the model is to produce caring acts that are committed to results, healing, promotion and protection. The greater the toolbox that workers use to shape care, the better they will be able to understand health problems and deal with them appropriately (MERHY, 2004; LIMA, 2001). Thus, Merhy and Lima's reflections point to the fact that the reorganization of work processes is a fundamental issue for changing the care model. In order to achieve this goal, it is essential to reverse the technologies used in the production of care, with a predominance of soft technologies that promote spaces of interaction between user and worker, with attention always directed at the user as the agent and central point of the process.

It is necessary for health workers to see themselves as doers of health acts and to present themselves as such in order to negotiate the proposed new model, to be recognized by the other individuals in the game and thus achieve legitimacy to act and contract (MERHY, 2003; LIMA, 2001).

Merhy (2003) emphasizes that health work is always linked to a humanitarian phase that must be incorporated into soft technologies, which form relationships and intercessions. The same author also asks us about the meaning of health work, from which it will be possible to understand all the dynamics inherent in the activities carried out in the context of Primary Health Care. In this sense, it is important for each professional to grasp and understand the actions they carry out on a daily basis, in order to establish an action policy that is consistent with the reality they are experiencing.

According to Campos,

> One of the main keys to ensuring quality in health would be an appropriate combination of professional autonomy with a certain degree of responsibility for workers. In other words, ways of managing would have to be invented that neither castrated workers' initiative nor left institutions totally at the mercy of the various professional associations. Autonomy presupposes freedom, but for autonomous work to be effective, it also presupposes the ability to take responsibility for the problems of others (CAMPOS, 2002, p. 232).

What we propose is the search for gains in autonomy on the part of the worker, considering that he or she is an active actor in the field of care production and that in the encounter with the user he or she is capable of triggering processes of mutual change and recognition, in the sense that every health worker is an agent of care and that every user is a protagonist in this process, to the extent that he or she brings a certain health need which, for us workers, represents a right to be legitimized.

2.3 THE HUMAN-WORK RELATIONSHIP AS A CONCEPTUAL TOOL FOR ANALYZING HEALTH WORK

It is well known that any job in itself is never neutral or aseptic; it always exerts an influence on the worker and on the work environment, producing instances that generate satisfaction or dissatisfaction, through the insertion of man in a relational field, of exchanges, of the development of "healthy subjectivities, of recognition and social valorization" (DEJOURS, 1992). In the author's view, the centrality of work suggests that it plays an essential role in shaping the public sphere, "because working is not just about producing: working is also about living together" (DEJOURS apud LANCMAN et al., 2008, p. 20). Work would be the main *place* where people learn democracy and the art of living together and establishing relationships, and would be conceptualized as an activity coordinated by individuals to confront what could not be achieved by simply carrying out a prescribed task, which requires an inventive, liberated worker capable of triggering processes of self-analysis, in the production of knowledge about themselves, and of self-management in the resumption of their singular know-how in the work situation in the molecular space (BAREMBLITT, 1996).

The meaning of free workers refers to the necessary openness that workers find within the organization of work so that they can take control of their production process, in other words, so that their subjectivity is constituted by a desire that motivates them to do something within the scope of the non-prescribed. Rolnik (2006, p. 96) warns us that this concept of freedom is different from that of "loose workers" who are more than free, but completely lost, which implies a "senseless crisis of subjectivity". The worker is deprived of his labor tools in the name of a production logic that doesn't match the reality of work, being more of a social character than an active agent of the activity he performs.

The worker, then, is a social character from the field of micropolitics, which according to Rolnik (2006, p.11) involves processes of subjectivation related to the political, social and cultural spheres, through which the "contours of reality are configured in their continuous movement of collective creation".

In the author's conception, the "micro" space constitutes the political component in which there are no units but intensities, immersed in a plane of non-subjectivized affections, determined by the agencies that the body makes in its immanent relationship with the world. In the space of micropolitics, a space of multiplicity, relationships permeated by power are inscribed, more precisely by the micro-powers produced in the confluence between bodies, which demystifies the idea of a social body constructed by units. Foucault (1993) states that power cannot be captured solely in the sense of ideology and that its ultimate nature is to be constituted where its intention is fully invested, in other words, within real and effective practices and in direct relation to its field of application. In reality, power is a tangle of relationships inscribed in an almost pyramidal and more or less coordinated structure. It is characterized as an open and strong system, in the sense that it exerts effects, whether positive or not, at the level of desire and knowledge, which refers to the fact that every relationship produced in the micro-space is inscribed by relations of power and regimes of truth production that determine the nature of relations between bodies that are in permanent struggle, delimiting certain territories of clash.

Every micro space is constitutive of a larger space, the macro, molar space, which for Institutional Analysis would be immanent to the molecular, establishing a mutual relationship of belonging. Macropolitics allows visibility, it is the only field that can be captured with the naked eye, having objective, enunciable forms that are constructed by unity and totality. It is the place of order, stability, precise limits, regularity, reproduction and conservation. Baremblitt (1996, p. 45) suggests that "the great historical changes, the macro-changes, are always the result of small changes and that the great powers that prevail in society are only forms resulting from small powers that collide and connect in microscopic spaces". The micro, molecular space would be the place of production, of the emergence of the new, the random, the unpredictable, the unthinkable, the emanation of the movements of desire. It is in the molecular space, of micropolitics, that micro-powers and the instituting movements of desire and subjectivity are inscribed, composing a plane of affections that are inherent to the relationship that is established between bodies in interaction with the individual/work instance, in other words, analytically, micropolitics would be understood as the "daily action of subjects, in the relationship between themselves and in the scenario in which they find themselves" (FRANCO, 2006, p. 1). These instituting movements in the composition of the encounters that take place in the "daily actions of subjects" are seen as a process, with a dynamism that allows them to transform institutions, constituting codes and signs that re-signify the relationship between the subject and the space of practices in which they are situated (BAREMBLITT, 1996).

The encounters that take place in molecular space are mediated by affects and intensities, in the sense that each body represents an essence, a degree of potency that allows this body to affect or be affected. Spinoza (apud Deleuze, 2002) distinguishes between two types of affect: appetites, which derive from the essence of the individual affected, and passions, which derive from the outside. For the Theory of Affections[1] , when we find a body outside our own that suits us, in other words, that is capable of increasing our power to act as relationships are formed, the passions that affect us are those of joy and satisfaction. On the other hand, when our body meets a body that doesn't suit us, its potency opposes ours, causing a subtraction or annulment, diminishing or eliminating our potency to act, giving rise to sad passions; we feel impotent since sad passions are always impotence.

The idea of the body from Spinoza's perspective does not conceptualize a body

---

[1] When we look at the theory of affect, it is essential to be clear about the idea of affect and affection, in the sense that affections are bodily marks or images, referring directly to the body, to a state of the affected body and implying the presence of the affecting body; Affect, on the other hand, refers to the spirit and represents for both the body and the spirit an increase or decrease in the power to act, more precisely the transition from one state to another (DELEUZE, 2002, p. 55 and 55). 55 e 56).

by its organs or functions, and "neither is a body defined as a substance or a subject", it is defined by the affections of which it is capable. Thus,

> A body, no matter how small, always contains an infinity of particles: it is the relationships of rest and movement, of speeds and slownesses between particles that define a body, the individuality of a body [...] and this power to affect and be affected that also defines a body in its individuality (DELEUZE, 2002, p. 128).

The Spinoza body doesn't just refer to a human being or a material substance, but can also be seen as a theory, an idea, a soul, a sound body, a social body, a body of knowledge that materializes in relationships inscribed in planes of composition and decomposition. Thus, the body would be defined through the relationships it produces and establishes, above all through the affections it is capable of feeling and

issue. It would be defined by longitude and latitude, which make up its cartography. The former refers to the "set of relationships of speed and slowness, of rest and movement, between particles that compose it [...] between unformed elements". Latitude would be the set of affects that make up a body at any given moment, an anonymous force represented by the power to be affected. The latitude and longitude body is always in a process of recomposition, production and composition by individuals and collectivities (DELEUZE, 2002, p. 132). The body in the latitude dimension, of the waves and vibrations of affections, produces magnetic fields made up of forces attracting each other in movement and rest, speed and slowness, stops and rushes (ROLNIK, 2006).

Rolnik (2006, p. 32) warns us that understanding the space of magnetic fields, also considered planes of consistency, the space of the molecular plane in which micro-powers and different becomings are inscribed, requires the use of the vibrating eye, which is different from the retinal eye, limited to the visible, biological and susceptible to illness. The vibrating eye is capable of crossing the boundaries of what is visible and is the constitutive of a vibrating body, without organs, which represents all the capacity of our senses together. In the micro-space of the relationship between individuals and between them and the instance of work, we recognize that the retinal eye alone is not capable of grasping the nuances of affections, subjectivities, desires and powers that make up the relationships in this territory, This is done through the vibrating eye, which is capable of seeing the "plane of consistency", produced by encounters and affections, which projects the field of vision to the invisible and "knows that this composition is the effect of a series of imperceptible processes of simulation".

The immanence between the retinal eye and the vibrating eye brings us back to the realization that grasping and understanding the relationships that are built up in the workplace requires more than simple observation, it requires listening to those who carry out the work and a polycentric, in-depth look in order to capture the complexity of the relationships established. According to Dejours (apud LANCMAN et al., 2008, p. 35), "in order to grasp work in its complexity, it is necessary to understand and explain it beyond what can be seen and measured", and it is essential to consider the nature of the relationships it fosters. For this to be possible, it is necessary to use a "hybrid compound", made up of the union of the molar retinal eye with the molecular vibrating eye, because what we are trying to grasp is the movement that arises from the permanent and fruitful tension between flow and representation, in the sense that the flow of intensities escapes the plane of organization of territories, disorienting their cartographies, destabilizing their representations and, by "stopping" the flow, channeling the intensities, giving them meaning (ROLNIK, 2006, p. 67). 67).

Subjectivity, inscribed in the man-work relationship in the molecular scenario, will always have effects that are concrete and real, even if unseen. In this respect, Dejours (1994) presents some preliminary questions based on the fact that the worker's body cannot be considered a "human engine", since it represents the object of endogenous and exogenous excitations; the worker has a personal history inscribed in desires, aspirations, motivations and needs and; each worker has different defense strategies depending on their life history. Baremblitt (1996, p. 50) brings us the idea of singularity as constitutive of a unique being, based on the fact that what "matters is not the production of similarities or analogies between subjects, but the production of differences, the singularity of each subject produced in each place, at each moment". The same author mentions that in the generation of the new, of a singular, instituting, contingent, circumstantial and revolutionary subjectivity, there is a continuous process of "the production of a free, non-subjectified, primigenic, productive, revolutionary subjectivity, in which desire is realized in local, micro connections and is carried out by generating the new" (p. 51), not by maintaining the old.

We start from the assumption that all subjectivity is inscribed in desires and that subjectivity in the conception of Deleuze (2000) and Guatarri (2005) is inherent to the idea of "other", the individual as process and product, a procedural field of moving forces and forms that emerge from these forces. Barros (2008) states that the human being is formed by a collective, networked, dynamic, unfinished process. When we recognize this "other" as a process, Dejours (apud LANCMAN et al., 2008, p. 253) points out that when engaged in the work situation, the individual clashes with components of the objective and social world because they have a subjectivity inscribed in their being, expressed by expectations and desires/power in relation to the realization of themselves in the field of social work relations. Thus, Spinoza's concept of the body is referred here to the concept of the "other", an epistemic and implicated subject (MERHY, 2004) who experiences a real work situation and has an arsenal of knowledge that constitutes their work tools, which are produced[2] and reproduced in practice scenarios. Merhy (2001) also affirms the

[2] The term production is used in the sense attributed by Institutionalism, as "that which is processed, everything that exists, naturally, technically, subjectively and socially. It is permanent

need to try to understand subjects as in action, being constructed by the practices that define them as an identity, while at the same time re-signifying these same practices in their spaces of freedom.

Desire, as an instance in the process of producing psychosocial universes, presents a first moment described by Rolnik (2006, p. 31) as one in which there is an encounter between bodies that have the power to affect and be affected, generating a mixture of affects that are exteriorized by "masks", taking shape in materials of expression. Thus, the worker always operates in scenarios of signs that are conditioned by desires that are the motivator of the work and that produce affections and disaffections in the arena of production, which becomes part of the field of micropolitics. In this field, the author states that there are no units but intensities, a list of affects determined by the agencies that are produced and, therefore, inseparable from their relationships with the world. What is perpetuated is the multiplicity compared to a "rhizome", through the observation that "in this path nothing is fixed, nothing is origin, nothing is center, nothing is periphery, nothing is definitely anything" (p. 61).

The concept of rhizome, which comes from botany and is incorporated into Deleuze and Guattari's discourse, is used to glimpse the so-called open systems of connection that take place through various agencies, "producing new relational formations on which the *socius* is built, the social environment in which each person is inserted" (FRANCO, 2006, p. 1). According to Rolnik (2006, p. 61), what appears is a "substantive multiplicity, unpredictable and uncontrollable becoming [...] which constitutes the immanent plane of the diagram that the rhizome, in its nomadism, embodies". What remains is the idea of "plan" as a variable instance, in a continuous process of change, "always rearranged and recomposed by individuals and

generation, while not crystallizing; it is becoming, and metamorphosis [...] we would call it creation" (BAREMBLITT, 1996, p. 46).

collectivities".

Taking up the concept of desire as a device[3] , Baremblitt (1996, p. 49) brings it to the level of the unconscious, the "unconscious forces" as they are considered by psychoanalysis. However, the desire of psychoanalysis is always tied to the Oedipus complex, a desire that endures in family life, in the incestuous fantasies of the infantile unconscious and which is projected into social life with the same intensity and nature. We would then have a restitutive, fulfilling, vague desire, devoid of power. On the contrary, for Institutionalism, desire is immanent to production, it seeks to create the new, connections, the power of invention. It is constitutive of being a worker and represents a motivator for activity, in the sense that "the worst thing about normative constraints is the annulment of desire" (FRANCO, 2006, p. 4). Foucault sought to relate desire always to the instance of power, so that desire itself is also power, and is structured from it, which explains the creative and innovative power of the desiring being, the one who desires and establishes relationships of affection in the name of this same desire.

From the perspective of Work Psychodynamics, desire is based on the Freudian idea of a set of,

> "Signs of the first experiences of childhood satisfaction, it refers back to a past and an individual history. Desire is inscribed firstly in the past and in what is not current; secondly in the fictitious, the illusory and the phantasmatic; thirdly in the individual and the subjective" (DEJOURS, 1994, p. 36).

The object of desire is not something real. In this proposition, behavior is understood as something of infinite importance, being considered an "accessory instrument" of the desire-pleasure relationship. Dejours' conception of desire is similar to

---

[3] The device is synonymous with agency, and is always "at the service of production, desire, life, the new". It is capable of generating revolutionary events and transformations, producing the lines of flight of desire, production and freedom. It would be something capable of triggering processes of change (BAREMBLITT, 1996, p. 74).

that of psychoanalysis, but diverges from the institutionalist strand and the theses of schizoanalysis, whose object of study is the "lines of escape, schizo lines through which territories are dismantled" (ROLNIK, 2006, p. 71).

Deleuze and Guatarri (apud BAREMBLIT, 1996) propose an idea of desire not just in the sense of a force that drives the psyche, but rather a productive and creative force that promotes encounters and is linked to other animating forces of the social, historical and natural. It would essentially have a productive-revolutionary and non-restitutive character. They also state that in Schizoanalysis desire is introduced into the field of production and production into the field of desire. "It is a question of learning to think of a desire that is essentially productive and a production, in the broad sense, that can only be desirous" (p. 58).

The study of the relationship between the psychic component and work organization was innovated with the publications of Chistophe Dejours, who appropriated the concept of Work Psychodynamics to replace that of Work Psychopathology, thus privileging the study of normality over that of pathology, seeking to understand how workers maintain a certain psychic balance, even though they are subjected to destructive working conditions (JACQUES et al; 2002). Thus, suffering arises as a result of a blockage between the worker and the work organization itself, understood here as a social relationship that involves negotiations and compromises.

The blockage of the relationship between the individual and the work organization, which is expressed in the dichotomy between prescribed work, seen as a task, and real work, an activity, imprisons the worker who is, above all, a desiring being who is constantly trying to adapt to the work situation, which can be imprisoning or liberating. What happens is a "fragilization in an upward spiral", in which the greater the disorientation, the greater the vulnerability that is captured by the distribution centers of meanings and values that seek to legitimize supposed knowledge and actions. There is a loss of sensitivity in the vibrating body, weakening the creative power of desire, dampening autonomy through the "dampening of the creative gesture" (ROLNIK, 2006, p. 101).

Conceptually, the field of Work Psychodynamics is defined by Dejours (apud JACQUES, 2002) as that relating to suffering, its content and meaning, placing its investigation in the field of the infrapathological or pre-pathological. Thus, suffering is seen as an intermediate clinical space that marks the evolution of a conflict between psychic functioning and defense mechanisms on the one hand, and destabilizing organizational pressures on the other. This field of study can be defined as:

> The dynamic analysis of the psychic processes mobilized by the subject's confrontation with the reality of work. Dynamic means that the investigation takes as its center of gravity the conflicts that arise from the encounter between a subject with a unique history, pre-existing to this encounter, and a work situation whose characteristics are largely fixed independently of the subject's will (DEJOURS, 1994, p. 120).

Work is seen as a mediator between the unconscious and the social sphere, understood as a "continuum" that extends beyond a restricted space and influences other spheres of life. The individual's identity is constructed in the relationships that take place at work, which generate pleasure and/or displeasure through moments of recognition. When recognition is absent, this has an impact on the worker's daily life. In this way, work can be a space for identity development and/or a factor of wear and tear/suffering for the subject. The instance of pleasure is made up of processes of recognition and retribution on a scale of a symbolic nature. Work generates pleasure when it can be recognized, both by the worker who experiences their individual contribution and by the other workers who make up this scenario of practices, in a plural sense of capillarity and mutual belonging to the collective production process (DEJOURS, 2006).

According to Brant and Gomez (accessed August 14, 2008), suffering is something in the subjective sphere that differs according to each individual's experiences and ways of going through life. It depends on the meaning it takes on in time and space, as well as in the body it touches, producing something "beyond the pleasure principle". Thus, "the boundaries between suffering, non-suffering and suffering-pleasure are imprecise, and overlap in indiscernible, often ineffable layers". In suffering, the body is deprived of power, it becomes an aptitude, there is an inversion of energy and powers, which makes the relationship of subjection strict. "Active force tends to become a reactive force of conservation", the autonomy of the working being is lost, individuals are taken over by a "galloping process of deterritorialization" (ROLNIK, 2006, p. 107).

Drawing an analogy with the idea of the nomad, Merhy (verbal information) states that in the nomad the territory to be traversed is within him or herself, his or her subjectivity outlines the dimensions of this existential territory which can either be within the individual and part of his or her being and/or be a space of symbolic insertion in which encounters are configured as process and product. In the conformation of suffering, the nomadic worker who travels through different existential territories is faced with the deterritorialization of knowledge, actions, affections and intensities. He is deprived of the leading role in his work process, since he is at the mercy of events that imprison him and impose him on a prison-like, oppressive work that is capable of completely tying up the freedom expressed in the worker's subjectivity, masking the production of the operating desire and not annulling it, since desire is constitutive of being an individual and represents power as a sphere of production.

Dejours (1996) presents new ways of dealing with suffering at work through the development of collective, creative and innovative formations against the stifling of freedom. This is what the author calls subjective mobilization, based on creativity, made possible by opening up public spaces for collective discussion. What the author recognizes is that the very deterritorialization of the world of work resulting from productive restructuring brings with it a reheating of the worker's desire, which creates mechanisms, individual or collective defense strategies that keep them in scenes of joyful or sad passions. Rolnik (2006, p. 89) adds that with the intensification of deterritorialization, desire is heated up and people are more exposed to random encounters, to affecting and being affected in different directions and with different intensities, which materializes in an immense procedural potentiality.

Merhy (2002) proposes that living work, which is constructed in the context of real work seen as an activity and which involves creation and freedom, should be made up of creative practices that take place in the intercessory space, consisting of actions such as welcoming, bonding and problem-solving, calling them soft technologies, which should be increasingly expanded to the detriment of the large and medium expansion already carried out, respectively of hard and soft hard technologies.

For Dejours (1996, p. 170), this translates into opening up spaces for creativity. He states that "the transformation of suffering into initiative and creative mobilization depends fundamentally on the use of the word and a space for discussion where perplexities and opinions are made public". The process of belonging and identifying with work depends fundamentally on the relationships that are established in everyday life, so that subjects are constituted from the "gaze of the other"; we recognize ourselves in the relationship with the other based on differences and similarities; individual or social identity is produced in intersubjective relationships through exchanges of affections and; the individual constitutes his or her singularity in the midst of differences (DEJOURS, 2008).

One of the contrasts of psychodynamic theory consists fundamentally in the idea of the dehistoricized individual, in the sense that the methodology of the individual interview is criticized for highlighting aspects of the subject's personal life, such as family history, which are seen as insignificant since "this methodology leads to not giving significant value to the subject's material, social and professional situation [...]" (DEJOURS, 1994, p. 124). Dejours' main concern was to study the collective of workers because he considered that in the collective experience, the dynamics of work are shared and emerge onto the visible plane. What determines the analysis of work, in this current, is the plane of the visible, what the retinal eye can apprehend as the sense of the finite, the limited, the one-dimensional. He sought the depth of a theory based on a subject who desires loss and restitution, who is deprived of something still enigmatic and who has a capitalist subjectivity[4] that is hardened by the constraints of the centralized organization of work. What Dejours did not take into account was the fact that the retinal eye would not be able to fully grasp the real dynamics inscribed in work relations, which would inevitably not be visible to the naked eye.

Brant and Gomez (accessed August 14, 2008), when rethinking the psychodynamics of work, in order to discuss the transformation of suffering into illness, point out that it remains tied to the,

> Thermodynamic and biological models, inherited from Freudian psychoanalysis and ergonomics. This is evident when Dejours develops the economic approach to psychic functioning, based on the medical model. From this point of view, the manifestation of suffering is interpreted as the result of a weakening of workers' collective strategies and not as a consequence of work-related situations [...] even though it has made considerable efforts to advance knowledge of the health-work relationship, Dejours' psychodynamics still encounters some difficulties, especially when it uses concepts such as "psychic balance", "psychic energy" and "normality" in a vague and imprecise way to explain suffering. Thus, by polarizing it into pathogenic and creative, Dejours reproduces a long tradition that, from the birth of the clinic to the psychodynamics of work, transforms suffering into illness, providing theoretical elements that collaborate in the construction of the identity of the sick worker.

It's clear that psychodynamics carries rigid shades of psychoanalysis through its organicist approach to the phenomena of the world of work, despite the fact that Dejours was concerned with the study of normality and not just the study of pathologies arising from work. However, the study of suffering and pleasure is based on the relationship between the worker and the work organization, which gives the theory a space to initiate an exercise of thought as the production of cartographies, with the admittedly incipient search for a break with a traditional exercise of thought that is maintained and seen through representation, reproduction and totalizing reason. This is what we see in the redefinition of the great productive machines, the great machines of social control and the psychic instances that define the way we perceive the world" (GUATTARI; ROLNIK, 1986, p. 27). Dejours' field of study, with the transition from a theory of the Psychopathology of Work to the Psychodynamics of Work, based on the realization that suffering did not always turn into illness.

The analysis is based on the psychodynamics of the intersubjective processes mobilized by work situations. Thus, the collective and individual strategies of workers, contrary to what Brant and Gomes say, are built when workers are already in situations of organizational constraints seeking to exercise their freedom in the pursuit of "mental health", that is, psychodynamics places them in the experience of suffering, at the moment when the individual experiences it at work, before becoming ill, not justifying the fact that the fragility of these strategies is the only cause for the experience of suffering. In fact, there is no explicit order of causality, but it seems that these strategies are more a result of a constraining and suffering work environment than a matrix for its construction. Collective defense strategies, in turn, contribute to the cohesion of the work collective, based on the realization that "working is not just having an activity, but also living: living the experience of pressure, living in common, facing the resistance of reality, constructing the meaning of work, of the situation and of suffering" (DEJOURS, 2006, p. 103).

Suffering would be strictly linked to the blockage that prescribed work exerts on the worker's inventiveness, since according to Dejours (2008, p. 21) "work is the creation of the new, the unprecedented", and the necessary adjustments in the organization of prescribed work require initiative, inventiveness, creativity and "ingenuity". The idea of normality brought up by Dejours (2006) in Psychodynamics is the result of a composition between suffering and the struggle (individual and collective) against suffering at work. Thus, normality does not represent the absence of suffering, which allows us to say that there is a kind of "suffering" normality caused by the dynamics of suffering at work.

One of the great merits of the current is its concern with the real effects of suffering/pleasure on individuals' daily working lives, recognizing that these effects extend to life "outside work". One of the innovations was precisely to think of suffering as an instance of conflict between the autonomy of man and his knowledge-power in relation to the rigid structures of work organization that create a gap between work seen as real and work seen as prescribed, which brings with it the nuances of a social organization of work that has its foundations structured on the ideas of Taylorism and Fordism, as well as the imprisonment of the will/freedom of the worker to the detriment of the will of others, represented by the organization of work itself.

We believe that even in limiting and painful work situations, individuals are desirous and seek the consummation of real work, living work, which is responsible for the production of an identity built on the relationship of affection with the other. Thus, the concept of prescribed work and real work, which form the pillar of Dejours' theory, in this study dialogues with the theory of dead work and living work in the field of health. Dead work, as referring to the rigid structure of production, centered on machines and equipment and structured knowledge, would be the expression of prescribed work, as it represents the standardization of the work process, essentially represented by the organization of work that constitutes the imposition of the will of others on the daily actions of the subjects. On the other hand, real work, which is produced in the freedom of the worker to re-signify his activity, would be the composition of living work, which in the field of health is work that is carried out in act, produced at the very moment it is consumed and conforms to the subject's power to act, a desiring subject who "desires to be, positively desires to exist, to be the world and part of it, desires as a will of 'power to be', as a desiring machine" (MERHY, 2007, p. 88). Just as prescribed work captures the worker in the space of intercession with real work, dead work also captures living work in act "in such a way that the worker may not be able to exercise any action autonomously, thus becoming completely bound by the logic of dead work" (p. 85), which can generate a "crystallization of living work into dead work", which is expressed in the diminution or annulment of the worker's power to act, which is at the mercy of encounters that decompose him.

In his analysis of health work, Merhy (2007) refers to it as being constituted by the encounters that take place between the worker and the user, creating an "intercessory space", which also exists in the worker/worker and worker/work organization relationships. This space, expressed here as a magnetic field (Rolnik, 2006), forms desiring forces and micro-powers that interrelate through intentionalities, subjectivities and agency that make up the encounters which are often conflictual and which determine the nature of the relationships built up in the subjects' daily working lives.

Merhy (1997; 2002) proposes that every health work process operates on the basis of "living work in act", which gives workers great freedom to act and their work an instituting power. This, combined with an intentionality centered on the ethics of care, is capable of bringing about changes in the way health care is produced, opening up processes of productive restructuring.

The idea of productive restructuring is attributed by Franco and Merhy (1999) as the novelties that emerge within productive systems that are capable of having an impact on the shaping of health work processes, being built on the basis of changes in the daily actions of the subjects at work. What remains is the realization that there is an "intentionality indicating the *modus operandi* that is unique to each individual. And the way of acting [...] has as an important device the processes of subjectivation that affect the subjects" in the sense that this same subject is imprinted with values and behaviors that are shared by the other subjects that make up the process.

When Merhy (2007) tells us about the toolbox that the worker has for carrying out his activity, he reveals that the command of living work over dead work is done, above all, through the tools that the worker has in his possession, so that:

> Living work cannot fully free itself from dead work within the work process, but it can control it if it learns to question it, to doubt its meaning and to open itself up to the noises/analyzers present in its daily life, With this, and in possession of a toolbox that is committed to the subject of the action, and in action, the logic of the work process, its management, organization and purpose can be reinvented, in act, collectively and publicly (MERHY, 2007, p. 71). 71).

Franco et al. (2006) state that there is a constitutive freedom of living work in act that is associated with the agency of desire, which is immanent to the activity of each worker, producing a "given social reality" that is inscribed in the world of work. In this way, work shapes a certain existential territory, in which an "ethical-political referential" operates, which workers adopt as a plane of consistency between themselves and the production of care.

Based on the freedom that constitutes living work in act, we believe that the experience of suffering at work is constructed at the very moment of the loss of this dimension of the freedom of know-how in everyday life, which exposes the subject to encounters that are produced in the multiplicity of established relationships and that generate passions of sadness, encounters of decomposition, generators of impotence. On the other hand, when this same freedom operates within the constraints of dead, established work, there is the perpetuation of the inventiveness and creativity of a working, desiring, powerful being, a passionate subject, an innate producer of compositions through relationships permeated by joyful passions that make up the field of pleasure at work, which occurs, above all, through the processes of mutual recognition of the collective belonging of subjects to the living and dynamic reality of the work instance.

2.4 THE WEB AND THE SPIDER: THE DAILY ACTIONS OF A WORKER AND HIS WEBS

According to Deluze (1987, p. 4), the word sign refers to the act of learning, so that signs are the object of learning, which is temporal and not abstract knowledge. Thus, learning would essentially be the act of considering an object, a being and a material as if they emitted signs that had to be deciphered and interpreted. The author uses the example of the carpenter and the doctor to say that the former is only a carpenter when he recognizes the signs inscribed in the wood, and the latter is only a doctor because he is able to identify a system of signs referring to diseases. In this way, "vocation is always a predestination in relation to signs".

What Deleuze suggests is that all the components of a given interpretative context are constituted and conformed through a multiplicity of signs that are singular, unique to each material or subject, so that "the unity of all worlds lies in the fact that they form systems of signs emitted by people, objects, materials; no truth is discovered, nothing is learned, if not by deciphering and interpreting" (DELEUZE, 1987, p. 5). However, this plurality of worlds consists of the fact that signs are not of the same type, cannot be deciphered in the same way and have different meanings.

The fact that we are sensitive to signs and see the world as something to be deciphered is a gift that could be hidden in us if we didn't have the necessary encounters. Thus, these systems are produced in the dynamics of affections that emerge from intersubjective encounters, which are full of different signs, meanings and desires that make up the scenarios of passions and affections described by Spinoza. The sign, in turn, would be the very essence of the individual, which enables them to affect and be affected in a state of permanent construction and deconstruction.

This discussion of the representativeness of the signs that emerge from the relationships between subjects leads us to think about the figure of the spider. But why a spider? Deleuze (1987, p. 182) uses the figure of this arthropod to exemplify what a body without organs is. According to the author, the spider "sees nothing, perceives nothing, remembers nothing. It just so happens that, at one end of its web, it registers the slightest vibration that spreads to its body in waves of great intensity and makes it, in one leap, hit the exact spot." Thus, the spider as a body without organs, the one described by Rolnik (2006) as the totality of the sense organs together, would be moved solely by signs that pass through its body like a wave and make it able to jump in search of prey, since "without eyes, without a nose, without a mouth, the spider responds solely to signs and is hit by the smallest of them". The signs, for the spider, would be its very essence, the essence of its very existence that drives it in multiple directions and between multiple senses, and they are what trigger the act of weaving with "each thread moving through this or that sign".

More than a body without organs, the spider, for us, is the figurative instance of an enviable architectural work, in the simple impulsive act of weaving its web. It would be the very essence of a job that is similar to the one that takes place in the daily routine of health work, based on the realization that a health worker, in this case the ACS, is constantly constructing his web, always operating in connective flows that bring about a cartography within the micropolitics of health work processes (FRANCO, 2006).

To begin this analysis, we turned to the biological characteristics of this spider. We started from the observation that a spider's webs are five times stronger than auger at the same diameter, can stretch four times their initial length and can withstand very low temperatures without breaking. The silk threads are produced by means of glands located in the abdomen, of which there are seven types that never occur in the same spider. The threads are used to encapsulate prey, form the frame, rays and spirals of the web and form cocoons. Another interesting fact is that many weaver spiders recycle their webs, which have to be renewed frequently. Observing a spider at work building its web, we can certainly see that there is an intrinsic wisdom in its technique: in the way it first extends the large support axis of the web and, from there, joins these support threads and fills the empty spaces with radial threads, quickly giving rise to a structure of impressive geometry, as well as great strength.

Understanding the web of a spider and its peculiarities, we look for the signs inherent in the act of weaving the web and transpose them to the work of CHWs. In this sense, the CHW in his daily activity, which constitutes a living work in act, is the builder of his web, a web that is unique to each individual and is characterized by its tenacity, resistance and elasticity, so that it extends over different territories, "capturing" actors who are part of the process and reconstituting itself according to the dynamics of daily work. This web is determined, in particular, by the encounters and agencies of which the CHA is capable, in the permanent construction of existential territories that form magnetic fields for the production of meanings and affections (ROLNIK, 2006).

What characterizes this web is its ability to renew itself, move around and build new connections. It would be a representation of the Rhizome, as it is made up of open systems that move through different territories and mobilize agents in the production of a *socius,* a social environment that is made up of the "lines of contact between social agents that are the source of the production of reality" (FRANCO, 2006, p. 1).

Thus, the work of the CHA is crossed by flows of intensities that emerge from the signs coming from the essence of the subject and those coming from the molecular space, which constitutes the field of the micropolitics of work, which is the result of a process that resurfaces within the CHA and triggers a production of life in itself, an autopoiesis seen as a "continuous production of itself, in which the living being preserves itself and continues to live in the realization of its individual ontogenetic history" (MATURANA, 1998, p. 200). Mariotti (1999) refers to *autopoiesis* by saying that *Poiesis* is a Greek term meaning production and autopoiesis means self-production. The word first appeared in international literature in 1974, in an article published by Varela, Maturana and Uribe, to define living beings as systems that continually produce themselves. These systems are autopoietic by definition, because they incessantly recompose their worn-out components. It can therefore be concluded that an autopoietic system is both producer and product and that they conform in circular directions, assuming a productive circularity.

Maturana (1998) emphasizes that all beings are immersed in an autopoietic system that is constituted as a unity, a network of producing components that in their interactions generate the same network that produces them, constituting its limits as part of it in its space of existence.

The ACS, as an innate builder of webs, builds them precisely in circularity, in the productive circularity described by Maturana, which allows connections in multiple directions. The intensities arising from the encounters that the agent makes operate at the heart of the system of signs inscribed in an autopoietic system of which he is a part, to the extent that he is capable of triggering within himself processes of producing life, of meaning, in such a way as to externalize his individual essence, represented as the power to act. Thus, when he is able to recognize himself as a potential essence in the production of life, he also allows himself to experience new encounters and affections, at the same time as he "captures in his web" new actors who are able to enhance the autopoietic system that constitutes the new silk threads, capable of spreading in new directions and meanings. Maturana (1998, p. 200) tells us about the very immanence between the subject and his circle of relationships, so that every being is in fact realized in a history of interactions, human beings being essentially social beings since "we live our daily being in continuous relationship with the being of others".

The silk threads that emerge from the autopoiesis inscribed in the ACS worker's being form a web that is characterized by diversity, production and breadth, forming geometrically from anchor points that are the very encounters that arise in everyday life. Schematically, the web of a CHW would be represented by the encounters of which he is capable:

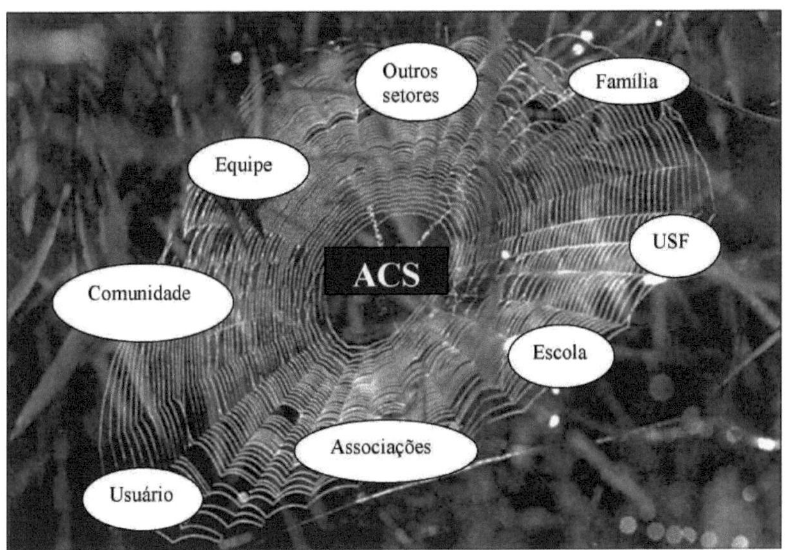

These encounters would be, above all, with users, communities, other team professionals, the USF institution, associations and other sectors that make up the space in which they work. However, when the CHW's work process is captured, i.e. when it ceases to be inventive, creative and autonomous, flaws appear in this web, ruptures that disrupt the relationships previously established and which, depending on the nature of the split, may not be able to be put back together again. The process of capture can occur by different means, whether it's due to the hegemony of dead work inscribed in hard and soft technologies (MERHY, 2002), or even through the disputes between the different nuclei of knowledge specific to each professional, which hegemonize practices that end up leaving the role that CHAs play in the day-to-day running of health services on the sidelines.

3 OBJECTIVES

3.1 GENERAL OBJECTIVE

To analyze the work process of the Community Health Agent of the Family Health Strategy in the municipality of Sao Gongalo/RJ, with a view to understanding the factors related to the production of joy and sadness in everyday work.

3.2 SPECIFIC OBJECTIVES

- Analyzing the work process of CHAs in ESF teams in the municipality of Sao Gongalo/RJ;
- Understand how the CHWs meet with the team and the community;
- Knowing the dynamics of sad and happy passions in the daily actions of CHWs;
- To identify the meaning of being a CHA for the subjects under study and what motivates them at work.

4 METHODOLOGICAL ASPECTS

Research in Public Health requires different approaches that necessarily follow interdisciplinary paths in which the incorporation of the human sciences as a theoretical-methodological resource has been fundamental in problematizing thematic fields and enriching their understanding.

The concept that reality does not exist as a ready-made totality that is external to the researcher, but rather as the researcher interprets it, highlights the compromised nature of this process and shows that the choices made go beyond merely technical aspects and are the result of the researcher's worldview (MINAYO, 2000).

In this way, the object of knowledge is cut out, delimited and defined based on the researcher's perspective of the reality in which they live, which, in turn, is the result of their historical and social positioning. Because of this, the object of social sciences is assumed to be intrinsically ideological, since it is impregnated by the researcher's worldview (MINAYO, 2000).

Bearing in mind that the most important element to guide the choices regarding the design of the study is the consistency between the methodology and the researcher's questions about the empirical reality, delimited as an object, in this research we opted for qualitative approaches, assuming the assumptions implicit in them, from the point of view of the researcher, a historically situated social subject.

This is the decisive stage of the research process. The problem for the researcher is not to capture a snapshot, like a photograph, but to catalyze the dynamics of the revelation-construction of the meaning of what is experienced and the dynamics of suffering/pleasure at work. In this way, the action of transformation involves mobilizing the subjects' capacity for analysis of their relationship with the work organization

(DEJOURS, 1994). The analysis of the subjective dimension of work necessarily involves access to the meaning that the situation has for the individuals themselves, and requires a reflexive work of collective elaboration guided by the desire for production and the will for emancipation of the participating workers (DEJOURS, 2008).

4.1 STUDY DESIGN

This investigation is an exploratory-descriptive, qualitative study that seeks to characterize and analyze the work of community health agents in Family Health teams, understanding how joy/sadness is produced in their daily work. Exploratory/descriptive research is a type of study that seeks to observe, describe and document aspects of a naturally occurring situation. It takes a qualitative approach based on the observation that knowledge about individuals is only possible by describing human experience as it is lived and defined by the actors themselves (LUNARDELO, 2004).

Qualitative health research works with the meanings of human supports, motivations, aspirations, beliefs, values, attitudes and relationships, apprehended from the point of view of the researcher, i.e. he captures a fragment or part of a reality. The emphasis is on understanding and analyzing the dynamics of the social relationships established through daily life and experience, understood within

structures and institutes (MINAYO, 1994).

Pope and Mays state that qualitative research,

> It is concerned with the meanings that people attribute to their experiences of the social world and how people understand that world. It therefore tries to interpret social phenomena (interactions and behaviors) in terms of the meanings that people give them; because of this, it is commonly referred to as interpretive research. [It studies people in their natural environments and not in artificial or experimental environments (POPE; MAYS, 2005, p.16).

Thus, the proposed methodology is appropriate to the objectives of this investigation, since the health work process and the work of the CHAs are social processes mediated by objectivity and subjectivity, with the capacity to incorporate questions of meaning and intentionality as inherent in acts, relationships and social structures. This study aims to describe the work of CHWs in the reality of the ESF in Sao Gonpalo and seek to understand it from the perspective of social practices.

4.2 RESEARCH SCENARIO

Describing the research setting, i.e. the environment in which the service takes place, is of fundamental importance, since it influences the shaping of the subject's personality, problems and situations of existence (TRIVINOS, 1987).

The setting in which work processes are carried out, in the day-to-day life of institutions, is a space conducive to unveiling the conflicts and noises generated in the production of health actions, as well as revealing the "way of acting" of each health worker who has their own tools for building their relationship with the user in meeting their health needs. In this way, the analysis of this space, where knowledge, practices and subjectivities intersect, allows us to understand and comprehend the way in which health support is produced in each professional's knowledge nucleus and in the field of practices, in which the nuclei are formed in the production of encounters and affections.

For convenience reasons, the research was carried out at the Jardim Catarina Family Health Unit, in the municipality of Sao Gonpalo/RJ, which was chosen by the municipality's primary care manager because it had a well-structured team of CHAs who had been working there since 2001.

4.3 RESEARCH SUBJECTS

The guiding idea is that each interviewee constituted an indefinite sum of knowledge from countless contacts and apprenticeships, forming a cycle of circulation and appropriation of infinite knowledge, so that any discourse was the result of collectively established knowledge transformed by personal experiences.

All the community health agents of a selected USF team were invited and voluntarily agreed to take part in the survey and the data collection strategies.

According to Minayo (2000), an ideal sample in qualitative research is one that is capable of reflecting the whole in its many dimensions. In this way, the instrument was applied to a team in the chosen Family Health Unit, prioritizing those with a low turnover of workers, structured and complete, i.e. containing a doctor, nurse, nursing assistant, community health worker and dentist.

4.4 DATA COLLECTION

The research technique chosen to collect empirical data was the semi-structured interview, a procedure that allows us to obtain information contained in the speech of the actors through facts reported according to the reality experienced. The interview is characterized by verbal communication which reinforces the importance of language and the meaning of speech, and is useful as a means of collecting information on a given scientific topic (MINAYO, 2001). The researcher's role in this context is to discover what is significant in the interviewees' statements, their concerns, interpretations and worldviews.

The interview was based on a semi-structured script (APPENDIX A) covering the characterization of the subjects under study, the process of working in the ESF, conceptions of the subject, the meaning of the work, satisfaction, dissatisfaction, joys and sorrows in daily life, suggestions and challenges, among others.

Minayo points out that in qualitative research the interaction between the researcher and the subjects is essential: "The interview is not simply a data collection task, but always a situation of interaction, in which the information given by the subjects can be profoundly affected by the nature of their relationship with the interviewer" (MINAYO, apud GOLSALVES, 2005, p. 99). He considers that "the semi-structured and unstructured interview differ only in degree, because in fact no interaction, for research purposes, is completely open". It starts with the preparation of a script which serves as a guide for the researcher.

Trivinos favors the semi-structured interview because "[...] while it values the presence of the researcher, it offers all possible perspectives for the informant to achieve the necessary freedom and spontaneity, enriching the investigation" (TRIVINOS, 1987, p. 146). In line with this idea, Cahue (apud LUNARDELO, 2004) states that this type of interview is organized on the basis of the themes that are to be addressed during the interview. However, the questions are not designed with purely affirmative or negative answers in mind; what is sought is interaction, flexibility and reflection.

The interviews were carried out individually, at the respective professionals' place of work, and lasted as long as it took to complete all the items in the script. We chose to record the interviews, after the interviewees had given their consent, and they were later transcribed in strict accordance with the structure of the subjects' speeches, in order to preserve the reliability of the statements. During data collection, notes were made about the approach to the field and the participants, as well as what the recorder could not capture, leaving it up to the eyes and mind to record this important information, such as expressions of silence and body language. Thus, direct observation was carried out in which the researcher observed the reality and daily working life of the subject under study in order to highlight aspects that were sometimes hidden in the participants' speeches, recognizing that the element that makes observation germinate is otherness, in the sense that the researcher appropriates the researched's way of going about life, in this case, the work dynamics that imprison or liberate, and the ways of coping with suffering that are unique to each subject. Observation as an instrument of qualitative research,

> It implies the activity of a researcher who personally observes situations and behaviors in which he is interested, without reducing himself to knowing them only through the categories used by those who live in those situations (CHAPOULIE, 1993, p. 585).

In order to identify the dynamics involved in the daily work of CHAs, the researcher immersed himself in the work of the agents as a complementary method, through ethnographic observation over a four-week period in the research settings, subsequently recording the nuances of this daily life in a field diary, which played a complementary role in data analysis.

4.5 MATERIAL ANALYSIS

The socio-cultural context evident among the research subjects is present in every speech and attitude of the participants, so the analysis was based on the apprehension of the meanings apprehended in the interviews, based on discourse analysis based on a cartography.

As a method of study, discourse analysis reached its apogee at the end of the 1960s, with the call for the totality of a society's utterances to become the object of study, recognizing that discourse differs from speech, being not only the transmission of information, nor the simple act of saying; on the contrary, discourse evokes an exteriority to language, ideological and social

(CARNEIRO, RODRIGUES, 2007). Thus,

> We can say that discourse, taken as the object of Discourse Analysis, is not language, text or speech, but that it needs linguistic elements in order to have a material existence. By this, we mean that discourse implies an exteriority to language, is found in the social and involves issues of a nature that are not strictly linguistic. We are referring to the social and ideological aspects impregnated in words when they are uttered (FERNANDES, 2005, p. 20).

As we have seen, discourse is an object of study that has no defined boundaries. It is three-dimensional - it is at the intersection of the linguistic, the historical and the ideological. It was therefore inevitable for discourse analysis to break with the postulates of classical linguistics, since it defines itself as the linguistic study of the conditions of production of an utterance.

Hegemony is sustained by discourse. From this it is not difficult to come to the conclusion that "discourse is not simply what translates struggles or systems of domination, but what is fought for, and the power we want to seize", as Foucault would say (1999, p. 10). Taking the floor is never a naïve gesture, as it is always linked to power relations.

One of the characteristics of this type of analysis is the concern with the "orientation of action", or the orientation of the function of discourse, which is seen here as a social practice. Language is seen as a practice in itself, based on an interpretative context in which individuals are inserted and on which they construct different discourses (BAUER; GASKELL, 2003).

As a first methodological requirement, we have the transcription of the interview data, which must be done in detail, not synthesizing the speech or correcting it. The data must be recorded reliably, preserving the richness of the accounts, based on the idea that "often, some of the most illuminating analytical institutes appear during transcription, because a deep engagement with the material is necessary to produce a good transcription" (POTTER apud BAUER; GASKELL, 2003, p. 252).

Transcribing the interviews evokes a spirit of skeptical reading, in which we have to question our own assumptions and the way we make sense of things in order to build an analytical mindset. In this way, it is possible to code the data, organizing the categories of interest, which allows the analysis to begin as such.

The discourse analysis was based on the cartographic method, since as a research method, "cartography provokes both analysis and intervention, since it affects the research subjects themselves and in this sense causes changes in their subjective constitution, and consequently, in their perception and action on reality" (FRANCO et al., 2006, p. 7). It is a method that reveals the processes of production of reality, highlighting its daily tension of "capture and freedom, through which plans for the production of life are formed, in movements of creation and invention, which would represent the new, as an expression of the agency of desire".

According to Kastrup (apud FRANCO, 2006, p. 7),

> Cartography is a method formulated by G. Deleuze and F. Guattari (1995). Guattari (1995) which aims to follow a process, rather than represent an object. In general terms, it is always about investigating a production process. From the outset, the idea of developing the cartographic method for use in field research in the study of subjectivity is far from the objective
>
> of defining a set of abstract rules to be applied. It does not seek to establish a linear path to an end. Cartography is always an ad hoc method.

Rolnik (2006, p. 23) points out that unlike a map, which always represents a static whole, cartography is a drawing that accompanies and is constructed with the transformational movements of psychosocial landscapes. Thus, "it accompanies and is made at the same time as the dismantling of certain worlds - their loss of meaning - and the formation of others: worlds that are created to express contemporary affections, in relation to which the existing universes become obsolete".

In this study, the cartographic method, as an analyzer of the marks of the encounters that are constituted in the relationships between the subjects, allows us to highlight the dynamics of the encounters experienced and constructed by the agents under study, in the sense of glimpsing the nature of the affections that are composed and decomposed in the daily work of the ACS.

To begin the analysis, we carried out a content evaluation based on the full transcription of the speeches and an exhaustive reading of the empirical material. To organize the data obtained, we read and reread the accounts, organizing and summarizing them in order to grasp the most relevant aspects, the phrases that are repeated or that stand out, thus seeking regularity.

Initially, the reports were grouped according to similarity, based on clippings and the extraction of relevant ideas, and the speeches were grouped according to familiarity. The Community Agents were referred to by the letter A followed by a number in order to guarantee the anonymity of the subjects under study.

4.6 ETHICAL ASPECTS

As all research with human beings involves a potential risk, be it moral or physical, it is essential to adopt measures that seek to safeguard the rights and duties of both research subjects and researchers in situations that may involve possible ethical conflicts.

At the beginning of the study, the consent of the Ethics Committee of the Fluminense Federal University was requested, in accordance with Resolution 196/96 of the National Health Council, which establishes guidelines and norms regulating research involving human beings. The study was approved by the Ethics Committee of the Universidade Federal Fluminense on February 13, 2009 under CAAE No.^{0} 46900000258-08 (ANNEX A).

Particularly in this study, the most relevant ethical aspect is that resulting from the interview situation, in which the participants talk about aspects of their life, their family and their relationship with the service provider, which may expose them to situations of vulnerability.

The adoption of measures that guarantee the anonymity of interviewees can protect them from this situation:

- Fictitious names were used for the participants when transcribing the interviews;

Omission of the use of any name of person, place or service that can serve as a reference to identify them;

- Letters and numbers were used to identify the speeches of the participants in this work.

Another important aspect is that the participants were informed about the researcher's affiliation, the aims of the research, the methodology used, the uses to which the results will be put and the ways in which the knowledge acquired will be disseminated, the risks they are being subjected to and their rights (freedom to participate or not, freedom to refuse to answer a specific question, freedom to leave at any time). Thus, before the interviews began, the CHWs were presented with the objectives of the research by providing them with the Free and Informed Consent Form (APPENDIX B), being informed that all the data would be treated confidentially and that consent could be withdrawn at any time without any penalty or onus.

5 AN IN-DEPTH ANALYSIS OF BEING A DAILY COMMUNITY HEALTH WORKER

By situating work as a regime of knowledge production, in which there is the continuous production of working subjects who are in their essence desires, needs, interests in conjunction and conflicts, and who move through different territories inventing the world and inventing themselves, we recognize that the world of work is "creation and use of self, but also struggle and resistance to work and to self" (SANTOS; BARROS, 2007, p. 64). The protagonism of work as creation is governed by the subjectivity and constitutive subjectivities of each worker who operates their work process and recreates the work of others through the triad of knowledge, power and subjectivity, which are in permanent implication. In this sense, the search for the meaning of work and the understanding of the relationships that are established in the field of production must be based on the discourse and actions of each worker. This led us to ask the CHW worker what he understands as recognition of the profession, the agencies of which he is capable and the open systems of connections that constitute his actions as a health worker. The CHW profession was signified as transformation, information, closeness and solidarity, as A8 put it:

"I think that the role of the community agent is something extremely active, it ends up being a person who has a mission to transform, always has a mission to transform, to change and ends up being a great opinion maker. The role of the agent is to help the population within their needs" (A8).

The identity inscribed in the work of CHWs positions them as nomads, as they move through different territories of knowledge and practice, constructing and deconstructing subjectivities determined by the encounters between the different actors and which shape being a CHW as a movement, a movement of developing oneself

(DELEUZE, 2001). They recognize themselves as a "link" between users and the health team, based on the realization that they are part of a chain that keeps users and the team's professionals interconnected.

"I think the role of the agent is very important in the community, because you're the one who captures all the problems in the neighborhood and brings them to the team, to the doctor who works more in the unit than in the community; he's not as active as the community agent. The community agent is everything, he's the strongest link in the chain, if there's no community agent there's no way for the doctor and nurse to work" (A5).

The fact that CHWs recognize themselves as a "link in the chain" gives them a great responsibility in their day-to-day work to establish and maintain the bond between the team's professionals and the users, which does not depend essentially on their work, since the field of the micropolitics of work is constituted by the subjective production of the working subjects, who are essentially singular subjects, The idea of the CHA as a link in the chain brings with it a vision of the professional as a "carrier", an observer of the problems affecting the community who would have the task of reinterpreting the reality seen in the light of the health team's established knowledge.

Schraiber (apud SILVA; DALMASO, 2002) points out that the work of CHWs can be described from two points of view, since one of the poles refers to the figure of a 'messenger' and a mere channel of communication with the community, or, on the other hand, to being a 'reforming agent' capable of bringing about changes in user care. According to the author, there is a polar oscillation between the accumulated personal experiences that would be essential, and even sufficient, for the constitution of the ACS and, on the other hand, the technical mastery of certain health procedures that would guarantee a nuclear and institutional reform in the field of health.

A5 reinforces the solidarity and relational aspect of his work by creating a professional identity that is based on meeting the health needs of the community and on the encounters that mutually affect the actors involved:

"Being a community health worker is being there, day-to-day, you're inside people's homes trying to help in any way you can, and ease the burden of problems a little, showing people the way, teaching them their rights" (A5).

The concept of identity at work brings us back to the idea of the construction that the actors make in the context of their own actions, in other words, it symbolizes a perception based on both collective and individual expectations and motivations. Thus, identity at work operates based on elements of the actors' subjectivity, but also on the subjectivity and objectivity derived from the agents' life experiences (SILVA; DALMASO, 2002), reinforcing Dejours' (2008) view that the real organization of work is a product of social relations inscribed in diverse knowledge and distinct subjectivities. O

work plays a major role in the formation of identity in the sense that "It is from the gaze of others that we recognize ourselves in a process of searching for similarities and differences; it is everyday relationships that allow the construction of individual and social identity, based on material and affective exchanges, so that the subject, throughout his life, constitutes his singularity in the midst of differences" (LANCMANN, 2008, p. 340).

Motivation as a desire to remain in the profession was referred to in this study as the possibility of helping others, the building of bonds of friendship and the recognition that the work carried out is capable of triggering processes of self-care and re-signification on the part of the users, who are empowered by their own care and recognize in the CHA an agent of transformation and resolution.

"What motivates you is friendship, you end up getting involved with some cases and you really want to help, you want to be there giving a helping hand" (A1).

"What gives me pleasure is seeing people in need of medication, a consultation, a needy person in need of medication, it gives us strength to work, to be able to help"

(A2).

"The motivation I have today is the families I've known for eight years, so we end up having a bond of friendship, they motivate me to keep working" (A6).

The result of the work is the greatest motivation for the agents, based on the understanding that the other is also a desiring being, with the power to manage and affect, despite the failures interposed in the encounter between the community agent and the users and the community, as A8 tells us:

"Motivation doesn't come from the managers, it doesn't come from the structural model they've adopted, but from the population, because when you realize that a person you've followed, in my case it's ten years, and many children we've followed since they were little, that ends up being a great victory for me, it gives me great satisfaction to realize that people are healthy, have quality of life, are taking care of themselves" (A8).

During encounters with users and the community, the CHA recognizes different signs that are formed verbally or non-verbally and interprets them according to their subjectivity and perception at work. In other words, the interpretation of these signs determines the increase or decrease in the worker's power to act, in a way that enables them to affect and be affected in continuous processes of construction and deconstruction. The interpretation of certain signs emitted by users, such as a smile of satisfaction and gratitude, generates an instance of recognition which is capable of increasing the CHA's power to act through the establishment of a joyful, constructive and creative encounter which is capable of producing new signs which are also emitted by the worker and which, when interpreted by users, can generate affections which will determine joyful or sad encounters. Thus, the interpretation of a sign generated in the field of work production is related to the perception of each subject involved and depends on the confluence of knowledge and power, the latter being considered as a desire to perpetuate the new, as production and creation.

"The greatest satisfaction is when they recognize you, because not everyone recognizes your work. But some recognize it a lot, to the point of giving us gifts, I think it's recognition" (A1).

"The greatest satisfaction is when you manage to solve their problems, see that they are satisfied, see the gratitude, build friendships, see that the community is doing well, see the fruits of the work" (A15).

The "spider" CHA, as an innate builder of webs on which the field of the micropolitics of work operates, is then affected by the recognition that comes from the encounter with the community, experiencing an increase in its potency, expressed as desire and generating joyful passions, at the same time as it emits signs represented by the activities of caring for users, seeking resolution and satisfaction (DELEUZE, 1987). It exercises its sensitivity as a body without organs that is capable of apprehending the signs generated by the end of the silk thread that captures the user and the community, interpreting them and emitting new signs that are recognized by the users and that guarantee the cohesiveness of the web, as it maintains the productive circularity as a territory for the eruption of affections and passions.

The psychodynamics of work presents the image of a triangle with the aim of linking the instances of suffering, task and recognition, each on a vertice, seeking to understand the interrelationship between them in everyday work life. Thus, it recognizes that the working subject incessantly seeks recognition through the encounter between the subject and the collective, so that the search is relative to recognition by the collective of the singular subject. He points out that more than recognition, the worker is looking for something in the singular sphere that is related to his subjectivity and his *modus operandi,* which makes up a singular hybrid CHA, with diverse subjectivities that are continuously composed through processes of subjectivation and deconstruction of what is instituted (LANCMAN, 2008). Recognition comes to be seen in the productive circularity of a web constructed by the ACS and which captures diverse actors, so that it passes through the ends, mutually affecting the collective and the singular and maintaining the cohesion and tenacity of the silk threads. In this respect, recognition is expressed, according to Honneth (apud MENDONQA, 2008), as social esteem, exercised through values such as solidarity and related to the maintenance of self-esteem, which determines its impact on the established encounter.

The fact that CHWs consider recognition as a substrate for building joyful encounters with users and the community does not guarantee that they will emit signs that will be interpreted by others as care or responsibility, since the circularity of the affections produced depends on the subjectivity of the actors involved, This is clear from the imposition of domineering and controlling care by the professional on the community, in search of success in the field of the imaginary that is related to changing the user's life habits and the verticalization of knowledge considered to be truth that the CHW acquires from the other professionals in the team in the space of the health unit. The CHW can then act as a "knife sharpener", who, according to Barros (apud PINHEIRO; MATTOS, 2008, p.280), acts on the basis of a "complacent, microscopic and caring" attitude, and who exercises guardianship care, in which the other is seen as weak, deprived of their subjectivity. The ACS who sharpens knives is unveiled in the actions of a controlling and operative care, which is clear in A5's speech when she mentions the care she gives to hypertensive and diabetic users. However, CHAs do not always perceive guardianship care as a reduction in collective creation and the theory that guides their daily work constitutes, intentionally or not, a "regional system of struggles, an ethical-aesthetic-political stance, whose assumption delimits certain territories of conflict" (apud PINHEIRO; MATTOS, 2008, p.281).

"What makes me happy in my profession is taking a patient with uncontrolled blood pressure and bringing them to the unit, controlling their pressure. The biggest challenge is to control all hypertensive and diabetic patients, to make them understand that what we say must be followed" (A5).

The chaos in the web produced by CHWs in their daily lives comes from the processes of capturing their work, which represents the failures experienced in encounters that generate sad passions, in which the power to act as an instance of production and desire is diminished. In this study, CHAs relate failure to the detailing of their knowledge in relation to the instituted knowledge of the team, being left out of decision-making processes and recognizing the limitation of their know-how in the face of the diversity they encounter at work.

"The work of the agent doesn't come up because nobody values our work, I prefer to be on the street, when you work here inside there are different people, different thoughts. There's a lot of conflict, each person has their own work profile" (A5).

A3 blames the actual organization of the work for the difficulty in accessing the team, recognizing that the capture of live work by the rigidity of a centralizing management produces a breakdown in meetings with the team.

"I see the need for one day a week to stop and put the cards on the table, the doctor and the nurse don't have much time to get together, be together, talk to the team and put the cards on the table, do some tidying up" (A3).

The social valorization of medical work and the subjectivity of this professional within the scope of the ESF produces in the ACS the experience of failure and dissatisfaction and hinders access to this professional who is isolated in a field of historically well-defined knowledge that does not allow for the immersion of different types of knowledge, in other words, which does not recognize the core of knowledge inscribed in the work of the ACS. Merhy and Franco (2006) present us with the idea that the organization of health care has been anchored in a model of care centered on medical consultation, on medical knowledge that structures and determines the knowledge of others, with the production of care being linked to hard and soft-hard technologies and with the figure of the doctor as the core of the work that is carried out in the daily life of health services.

'Sometimes the doctor makes it difficult, there's that hierarchy, the community agent and the community agent and the doctor and the doctor. There are doctors who think the agent is nothing, I have a hard time dealing with that" (A2).

"He's like that, everything has to be the way he wants it, the way he wants it, I'm the doctor and I know what he needs, but we're the ones on the street and we know what his disabilities and difficulties are" (A4).

From this point of view, it is proposed to recognize the work done by and with other workers, acknowledging it as a constitutive part of collective health work. In reality, what exists is an unequal social valuation of the different jobs, which leads us to the inequality between the jobs performed, which translates into relations of power and hierarchy between workers in the various areas of activity. This hierarchy is linked to management, organizational structure, professional areas and different jobs, which generates relations of command and maintenance of the *status quo,* reproducing the technical-social division of modes of production (GALAVQTE, 2007). The limitations imposed by management and the organization of work itself have the effect of diminishing the CHW's power to act, generating sadness and stifling the worker's creativity and inventiveness. Barros (2007, p. 67) characterizes this process as an "amputation of the worker's initiative" which occurs through the silencing of creative movements.

"What makes our work difficult is the low number of appointments, the lack of medication, the lack of infrastructure. I want to do something, but what can I do? I can't do anything, I have no way of doing anything" (A6).

The reduction in the CHA's initiative in the encounter with work management translates into a limitation that deprives the worker of his own work process and makes it impossible for him to do anything in the realm of the non-prescribed, which makes us think of the power that prevails of dead work over living work and which leads to the loss of the dimension of freedom of know-how in everyday life, exposing the subject to encounters of decomposition, generating impotence.

"The biggest challenge is the lack of structure we have in terms of materials, there's not much to offer the person, what I say the most is: 'I can't, I don't have it, there's no medicine today'. I think we have the capacity to do more, to better serve the community, what we do here is make appointments" (A7).

Merhy (2003), in unraveling medical work, points out that valises represent technological toolboxes of knowledge and their material and non-material developments, which make sense according to the scenario in which they are produced and governed, and according to the encounters in which they operate. In this sense, the community worker operates, above all, in the field of relational valises, the production of affects and signs through a "working knowledge", which according to Mendes

Gongalves (apud SILVA; DALMASO, 2001) represents a break with scientific knowledge that cuts out the object of intervention and imprisons real, productive work. This instance of knowledge allows us to understand everyday practice as production and re-signification and operates, above all, through the encounters triggered between the actors involved. A2 highlights the main valises he uses as operative knowledge.

"Patience, love for them, understanding. We don't do it anymore because we can't" (A2).

"What I use most is dialog, speaking, listening, information, the knowledge I've acquired in my daily experience and in the training I've received" (A5).

The CHW's field of knowledge is built up based on the knowledge they acquire from working with the team's professionals, from the training they attend on related topics such as leprosy, tuberculosis, children's health, women's health, among others, and on the knowledge they bring with them from life experiences that are related to their subjectivity, which for Deleuze (2001) represents a double power as it believes and invents, presumes secret powers and assumes abstract, distinct powers.

"I've done a lot of courses, it's helped me a lot, dealing with people, understanding what the doctor says, what the nurse says, in the past we didn't understand, it's improved a lot. Now I work with the knowledge I bring from my life and the new knowledge I've acquired with the community and in the Unit" (A1).

The production of knowledge in the meeting with the health team is done in a vertical way, with the mere transmission of knowledge that can instrumentalize the CHA's daily actions, in other words, they absorb the discourse of the doctor and nurse and apply it in the meeting with the community. It is clear that the CHW is considered by the team to be a "blank page", so that the knowledge he brings from his life experiences does not find a place in a space of supremacy of biomedical knowledge that reproduces care centered on the field of hard and soft technologies described by Merhy (2002) as well-structured equipment and knowledge. The same author also reinforces the idea that health work can take on two scopes, i.e. on the one hand it can be centered on a prescriptive act that legitimizes a model centered on hegemonic medical knowledge, which produces knowledge, and on the other hand it can take the form of intercessory relationships established in live work and in act that produces care that generates gains in autonomy on the part of the user.

A6 recognizes the flaws in the process of producing knowledge in the meeting with the team's workers and says that "it's the experience on the street that makes you learn", since in the meeting with the community the CHA is able to manage their actions and exercise the creativity and inventiveness of their know-how, in other words, in the space of the community they are free to produce care and establish new encounters. In this respect, Merhy (2003) states that,

> All the actors involved in the production of health govern certain spheres, given the degree of freedom that exists in the daily actions of health work. This presupposes that the care model is always constituted on the basis of certain contractual arrangements between these social and political actors, even if this agreement takes place under strong tension, since the way in which care is organized is a product of it (MERHY, 2003).

For this analysis, psychodynamics comes into play by composing a worker as an operator and ruler of his real work, reinventing and recomposing his work in the midst of conflicts, especially those related to the organization and management of work processes. It is brought into the analysis of the work of CHAs by proposing the triangular and intercessory image between the instances of suffering, work and recognition that determine the construction of an identity at work, based on the realization that workers can experience different affects on a daily basis that will determine the impact of work on them, on the product and the 'consumed'C However, it is clear that the CHW, when composing his web of relationships, is exposed to the crossing of different signs and affects that are formed in a circular and continuous way and not just in a hierarchical way as in the pyramid. Thus, the study of the work of CHWs reveals the cartography of a web with connected lines that break and recompose themselves according to the nature of the encounter established and the affections that are composed in this cohesion.

6 FINAL CONSIDERATIONS

"There are moments in life when the question of whether one can think differently from what one thinks, and perceive differently from what one sees, is indispensable in order to continue looking or reflecting" (Michael Foucalt).

Unveiling the daily work of CHWs in this study reveals a worker who operates in molarity and plurality, a hybrid that permeates different territories of the triad of power, knowledge and subjectivity. What exists is a gap between the profile expected by the laws that regulate the profession and the real CHW, a singular protagonist in the field of work production. According to FERREIRA (2008, p. 45) "at times they may be more inclined to help in solidarity and at others less, or perhaps not at all, but this does not mean that this characteristic is inherent in the agent's subjectivity and that their presence is a condition for good encounters". Thus, the CHA profession is not based on vocation and solidarity if we consider that being a community worker is inscribed in a territory of conflicts, subjectivities, desires, micro-powers and that they operate, above all, on the basis of an interested view of reality. There is no way of defining a profile for CHAs, since they are workers who, like others, invent and reinvent their work processes on a daily basis. We should talk about subjectivity and not a profile, since we are talking about a polycentric worker who operates his own work process with a certain degree of freedom.

The cartography of the CHW's work revealed Deleuze's (1987) figure of the spider, since the CHW, like other health workers, provides care at the moment of the encounter with the user and the community, i.e. the work 83 which he performs is eminently relational, intercessory, and through his body without organs, expressed as perception and subjectivity, he is able to sense the signs emitted by the different actors and which, when interpreted, have the power to affect the ACS, increasing or decreasing his power to act, which leads him to emit signs that guarantee the firmness and cohesion of the web.

In the encounter with the user and their health needs, the CHW can operate a care-care, in which there are gains in autonomy on the part of the user, who is seen as a co-author in the field of work production, or manage a procedure-centered care, exercised through the use of hard and soft-hard technologies that plaster the other who is seen as passive, and who absorbs the imposed knowledge considering it to be truth. This gives rise to the image of the CHW as a knife sharpener, who imposes centralizing and dominating care on the other, which deprives the subject of their own inventiveness and autonomy. Thus, the CHW leaves the image of the oppressed/victim and assumes that of the oppressor, in other words, the worker with a so-called "profile" proposed in the laws leaves the scene and a desiring and singular worker emerges with intentions that are inscribed in the lines and flows that make up the field of the micropolitics of work. It is clear that the CHW is the protagonist of his work, which makes it naïve to consider him a victim of the constraints of a plastered job, which is actually also produced by him in his actions.

Schraiber (apud SILVA; DALMASO, 2002) that the lack of definition of the CHA's role makes it difficult to delimit their performance as a member of the health team institution, it is clear that the encounters that generate sadness are experienced, especially in the relationship with the team's professionals and the work management itself, which end up breaking the web that the CHA weaves in their daily actions and which, once recomposed, ends up presenting grooves and scars that redirect the nature of the established encounter. The grooves represent the lines of escape which, according to FERREIRA (2008, p. 44)

> "they serve as devices for different agencies [...] the worker may or may not have an identity with the community, be in solidarity or not, serve more or less as a mediator depending on how the processes of subjectivation have occurred in their life and how much they allow their affections to pass, that is, the threshold of deterritorialization they can withstand".

As a point of consideration, we can look at the confluence of two concepts presented by Deleuze (2002), that of "good or bad", which characterize the polarity we find in the work of CHAs and in the encounters they establish. For the author, a good or strong person is one who is capable of organizing encounters, of joining in with what suits them and who is capable of increasing their potency, since this goodness has to do with dynamism, the composition of potencies. On the other hand, the bad or weak person is the one who lives at the chance of encounters, passively suffering the consequences and continually having their reduced potency revealed. In this way, we are faced with a CHA who moves between the good and the bad, who permeates different territories and who is able to direct the encounters, managing his work process, which removes the idea of victimization of this worker in the face of the capture of his work by the instituted knowledge of the team or even by the rigidity of work organization. We can also consider the possibility of the same CHW bringing together these divergent characteristics, at different times, which at first seem contradictory, but express the multiple being that he is.

Thus, CHAs are not homogeneous in the way they think and act in health care. There are those who operate according to care-care practices, welcoming and establishing bonds with users; and those who have a care-not-care practice, because they are centered on the idea that associates care with procedure. This diversity greatly characterizes the daily actions of CHAs, making it impossible to generalize their conduct, since it should be seen as a range of possible user care practices.

Indefiniteness is one of the most profound experiences in the daily work of CHWs, not just because they are not given a body of well-defined knowledge a *priori*, but because their work is constituted in plurality, in the most diverse and tenuous encounters, in which they affect and are affected by different passions. The work of CHWs is in itself potency, diversity, indefiniteness, search, ruptures, contractualities and escapes. The work of CHWs is, by its very nature, a conflict with oneself and with others.

7 REFERENCES

ALEIXO, J. L. M. Atengao Primaria a Saude e o Programa de Saude da Familia: perspectivas de desenvolvimento no início do terceiro milenio. **Revista Mineira de Saude Publica**, Belo Horizonte: v. 1, n. 1, p. 1-16, jan./jun. 2002.

ALMEIDA, M. C.; MISHIMA, S. M. The challenge of teamwork in Family Health Care: building "new autonomies" at work. **Interface- Comunicagao, Saude, Educagao,** Botucatu, v. 9, 2001. Available at: <http: //www.scielo.br.htm.>. Accessed on: June 20, 2006.

BAPTISTA, L. A. A **cidade dos sabios**: reflexoes sobre a dinamica social nas grandes cidades. Sao Paulo: Summus, 1999.

BAREMBLITT, G. **Compendium of Institutional Analysis and other currents**: theory and practice. 3. ed. Rio de Janeiro: Rosa dos Tempos, 1996.

BARROS, M. E. B. From knife sharpeners to cartographers: the activity of care. In: PINHEIRO, R.; MATTOS, R. A. (org). **Caring for care**: responsibility for the integrality of health actions. Rio de Janeiro: LAPPIS, 2008.

BARROS, M. E. B. From knife sharpeners to cartographers: the activity of care. In: PINHEIRO, R.; MATTOS, R. A. (Org). **Caring for care**: responsibility for the integrality of health actions. Rio de Janeiro: LAPPIS, 2008, p. 279-295.

BAUER, M. W.; GASKELL, G. **Qualitative research with text, image and sound**. 2. ed. Petropolis: Vozes, 2003.

BORGES, I. H.; MOULIN, M. G.; ARAUJO, M. D. **Organización do Trabalho em Saude:** multiplas dimensões. Vitoria: UFES, 2001.

BOSI, M.L.; UCHIMURA, K. Y. Quality evaluation or qualitative evaluation of health care? **Revista de Saude Publica**, Rio de Janeiro, v. 41, n. 1, 2007. Available at: <http: //www.scielo.br/>. Accessed on: June 2, 2007.

BRANT, L. C.; GOMEZ, C. M. **The transformation of suffering and illness**: from the birth of the clinic to the psychodynamics of work. [n.d.]. Available at: http: <//www.interfaz.com.br/transfsofrimen. />. Accessed on: August 14, 2008.

BRAZIL, National Council of Health Secretaries. **Monitoring and evaluation of primary care**. Brasilia: Conass, 2004. Available at: < http: //www.conass.com.br/paginas/conass_documenta.php//>. Accessed on: July 20, 2005.

BRAZIL, Ministry of Health and Pan American Health Organization. **25 Years of Alma-Ata:** Health and the Right of All. 2003. Available at: <http://www.opas.org.br/>. Accessed on: November 1, 2005.

BRAZIL. Law 10507, of June 10, 2002. Creates the profession of Community Health Agent and makes other provisions. **Diario Oficial [da] Republica Federativa do** Brasil, Brasilia, June 10, 2002.

BRAZIL. Ministry of Health. **Programs and Projects - Family Health**. Available at: <http: //www.saude.gov.br//>. Accessed on: July 3, 2005.

BRASIL. Norma Operacional Basica do Sistema Unico de Saude-NOB-SUS 01/96. **Diario Oficial [da] Republica Federativa do** Brasil, Brasilia, November 6, 1996.

BRAZIL. Ordinance No. 1886/GM, of December 18, 1997. Approves the Norms and Guidelines for the Community Health Agents Program and the Family Health. **Diario Oficial [da] Republica Federativa do** Brasil, Brasilia, December 18, 1997.

BRAZIL. Ordinance No. 648, of March 28, 2006. Approves the National Primary Care Policy, establishing revised guidelines and norms for the organization of Primary Care for the Family Health Program (PSF) and the Community Health Agents Program (PACS). **Diario Oficial [da] Republica Federativa do Brasil**, Brasilia, March 28, 2006.

BRITO, J. C. Health work: looking at and experiencing the SUS in everyday life. **Cad. Saude Publica**, Rio de Janeiro, v.21, n.5, sept./oct. 2005. Available at: <http://www.scielo.br/scielo.php />. Accessed on: July 20, 2005.

CAMPOS, C. E. A. The challenge of comprehensiveness from the perspectives of health surveillance and family health. **Cienc. Saude Coletiva**, Rio de Janeiro, v.8, n.2, Jan/.2003. Available at: <http://www.scielo.br//>. Accessed on: July 20, 2005.

CAMPOS, F. E.; BELISARIO, S.A. The Family Health Program and the challenges for professional training and continuing education. **Interface- Communication, Health and Education**. Botucatu: n. 9, August 2001.

CAMPOS, G. W. S. **A method for analyzing and co-managing collectives**: the constitution of the subject, the production of use value and democracy in institutions: the wheel method. Sao Paulo: Hucitec, 2002.

CAPISTRANO, D. Filho. **Health and cities**. Sao Paulo: Hucitec, 1995.

CARNEIRO, E. A.; RODRIGUES, E. C. A. Introductory notes on discourse analysis. 2007. Available at: http://www.artigos.com/artigos/filosofia/. Accessed on: September 20, 2008.

CARVALHO, V.L.M. A **Pratica do Agente Comunitario de Saude**: um estudo sobre sua dinâmica social no município de Itapecerica da Serra. 2002. 150f. Dissertation (Master's Degree)-Faculty of Public Health, University of Sao Paulo, 2002.

CASATE, J. C.; CORREA, A. K. Humanization of health care: knowledge conveyed in the Brazilian nursing literature. **Rev. Latino-Am. Enfermagem**, Ribeirao Preto, v.13, n.1, jan./feb. 2005.

CHAPOULIE, J. M. **La place de l' observation et du travail de terrain dans la recherche en sciences sociales**. Actes du colloque du Conseil Quebecois de la Recherche Sociale de l'Acfas, 1993, p. 67-82.

CLOT, Y. **A funpao psicologica do trabalho**. 2. ed. Rio de Janeiro: Vozes, 2007.

COHN, A.; MARSIGLIA, R. G. Process and organization of work. In: ROCHA, L. E. et al. (Org). **Is this people's work**? Sao Paulo: Vozes, 1993, p. 56-75.

CONTANDRIOPOULOS, A. P. Evaluating the institutionalization of evaluation. **Cienc. Saude Coletiva**, Rio de Janeiro, v.11, n. 3, p.705-711, 2006. Available at: <http://www.scielo.br//>. Accessed on: May 10, 2007.

CORDEIRO, H. O PSF como estrategia de mudanga do modelo assistencial do SUS. **Cadernos de Saude da Familia**, Brasilia, year 1, n. 1, p. 13-18, 1996. Available at: <http: //www.scielo.br//>. Accessed on: June 2, 2006.

CREVELIM, M. A. Community **participation** in the family health team: is it possible to establish a common project between workers and users? **Cienc. Saude Coletiva**, Rio de Janeiro, v.10, n.2 [cited November 14, 2005], p.323-331, abr./jun. 2005. Available at: <http://www.scielo.br//>. Accessed on: July 10, 2005.

DEJOURS, C. **The trivialization of social injustice**. 7. ed. Rio de Janeiro: FGV, 2006.

DEJOURS, C. **The madness of work**: a study in the psychopathology of work. 5. ed. Sao Paulo: Cortez-Obore, 1992.

DEJOURS, C. **Psicodinamica do trabalho**: contribuigoes da escola dejouriana a analise da relagao prazer, sofrimento e trabalho. Sao Paulo: Atlas, 1994.

DEJOURS, C. A new vision of human suffering in organizations. In: CHANLAT, J. **O individuo na organizagao**. Sao Paulo: Atlas, 1996.

DELEUZE, G. **Empiricism and Subjectivity**: an essay on human nature according to

Hume. Sao Paulo: 34, 2001.

DELEUZE, G. **Espinosa**: practical philosophy. Sao Paulo: Escuta, 2002.

DELEUZE, G. **Proust and the signs**. Rio de Janeiro: Forense Universitaria, 1987.

FERRAZ, L.; AERTS, D. R. **O cotidiano de trabalho do agente comunitario de saude no PSF em Porto Alegre.** Available at: <//http: www.scielo.br/. Accessed: June 10, 2006.

FERREIRA, V. S. C. **Micropolitica do Processo de Trabalho do Agente Comunitario de Saude: territorio de produgao de cuidado e subjetividades**. 2008. Thesis (Doctorate)-Postgraduate Program in Clinical Medicine, Federal University of Rio de Janeiro, Rio de Janeiro, 2008.

FOUCAULT, M. **Microfisica do poder**. 11. ed. Sao Paulo: Graal, 1993.

FRANCO, T. B. Networks in the micropolitics of the health work process. In: PINHEIRO, R.; MATTOS, R. A. (Org). **Management in networks**: evaluation, training and participation practices in health. Rio de Janeiro: ABRASCO, 2006.

FRANCO, T. B. et al. **The subjective production of the Family Health Strategy,** in Franco, T.B. et AL (eds.); The Subjective Production of Care: cartographies of the Family Health Strategy. Hucitec, Sao Paulo, 2009 (170 pages).

FRANCO, T. B.; BUENO, W. S.; MERHY, E. E. O acolhimento e os processos de trabalho em saude: o caso de Betim (MG). In: MERHY et al. **O trabalho em saude**: olhando e experenciando o SUS no cotidiano. Sao Paulo: Hucitec, 2003, p. 37-54.

FRANCO, T. B.; MERHY, E. **PSF**: contradictions and new challenges. Belo Horizonte/ Campinas, March 1999. Available at: <http://www.datasus.gov.br/cns/cns.htm/>. Accessed on: November 1, 2005.

FRANCO, T. B.; PERES, M. A.; FOSCHIEIRA, M. M. **Acolher Chapeco:** uma experiencia de mudanpa do modelo assistencial, com base no processo de trabalho. Sao Paulo: Hucitec, 2004.

GALAVOTE, H. S. Desvendando os processos de trabalho do agente comunitario de saude nos cenarios revelados na Estrategia Saude da Familia no municipio de Vitoria. **Ciencia & Saude Coletiva**, on-line, 2007. Available at: <http://www.cienciaesaudecoletiva.com.br/>. Accessed on: October 7, 2008.

GONSALVES, Elda M. Borges. **The Dental Surgeon's Work Process in the Family Health Program:** a contribution to the construction of the SUS. 2005, 140 f. Dissertation (Master's) - Postgraduate Program in Collective Health Care, Health Sciences Center, Federal University of Espirito Santo, 2005.

GUATTARI, F.; ROLNIK, S. **Micropolitica**: cartografias do desejo. 2. ed. Petropolis, 1986.

GUATTARI, F.; ROLNIK, S. **Micropolitica**: cartografias do desejo. Petropolis: Vozes, 2005.

HOLANDA. A. F**. - Dialogue and Psychotherapy**: correlations between Carls Rogers and Martin Buber. Sao Paulo: Lemos Editorial, 1998.

JACQUES, M. G.; CODO, W. **Mental health and work**: readings. Petropolis: Vozes, 2002.

LANCMAN, S.; SZNELWAR, L. I. (org). **Christophe Dejours**: da psicopatologia a psicodinamica do trabalho. 2. ed. ampliada. Rio de Janeiro: Fiocruz, 2008.

LERVOLINO, S. A.; PELICIONI, M.C. F. The use of focus groups as a qualitative methodology in health promotion. **Rev Esc Enf USP**, v. 35, p. 115-21, jun 2001.

LEVCOVITZ, E; MACHADO, C. V.; LIMA, L. D. A. Health policies in the 1990s: intergovernmental relations and the role of basic operational standards. **Ciencia e**

Saude Coletiva. Rio de Janeiro, v. 6, n. 2, p. 269-291,2002.

LEVORLINO, S. A.; PELICIONI, M. C. F. **The use of focus groups as a qualitative methodology in health promotion**. 2001. Available at: http:<//www.ee.usp.br/>. Accessed on: September 20, 2008.

LEVY, F. M.; MATOS, P. E. S., TOMITA, N. E. **Community health agents program**: the perception of users and health workers. Cad. Saude Publica, Rio de Janeiro, v. 20, n. 1, p. 197-203, 2004.

LIMA, R. and C. D. **Enfermeira**: uma protagonista que produz cuidado no cotidiano do trabalho em saúde. Vitoria: Edufes, 2001

LUNARDELO, S. R. **O Trabalho do Agente Comunitario de Saude nos Nucleos de Saude da Familia em Ribeirao Preto/Sao Paulo.** 2004. 156 f. Dissertation (Master's Degree)-Postgraduate Program in Public Health Nursing, University of Sao Paulo, Ribeirao Preto, 2004.

MARIOTTI, H. **Autopoiesis, culture and society**. [n.d.]. Available at: http:<//www.geocities.com/pluriversu/autopoies.html/>. Accessed on: August 20, 2008.

MARTINES, W. R. V.; CHAVES, E. C. Vulnerability and suffering in the work of the community health agent in the Family Health Program. **Rev. Esc. Enferm. USP**, Sao Paulo, v. 41, n. 3, p. 426-33, 2007.

MARX, K. **Capital**. 7. abridged ed. Rio de Janeiro: Zahar editores, 1982.

MARX, K. **Capital**. Sao Paulo: Nova Cultura, v. 1, 1996.

MATURANA, H. R. **Da biologia a psicologia**. 3. ed. Porto Alegre: Artes Medicas, 1998.

MENDES, Eugenio V. **The Great Dilemmas of the SUS**. Salvador: Casa da Saude, 2001.

MENDONQA, P. E. X. **(LUTA) In defense of life: tension and conflict, recognition**

and disrespect in the management practices of the Unified Health System. 2008. 143 f. Dissertation (Master's) - Postgraduate Program in Clinical Medicine, Federal University of Rio de Janeiro, Rio de Janeiro, 2008.

MERHY, E. E. (org). **Health work**: looking at and experiencing the SUS in everyday life. Sao Paulo: Hucitec, 2003.

MERHY, E. E. In search of lost time: the micropolitics of living work in health. In: MERHY, E. E.; ONOCKO, R. (Org). **Acting in health**: a challenge for the public. 3. ed. Sao Paulo: Hucitec, 2007, p. 71-112.

MERHY, E. E. *et. al.* Perspective of regulation in supplementary health in the face of care models. **Ciencia e Saude Coletiva**, Rio de Janeiro, v. 9, n. 2, p. 433444, abr/jun. 2004.

MERHY, E. E. In the Institutes, no one is powerless: preface. In: LIMA, R. C. D. **Enfermeira**: uma protagonista que produz o cuidado no cotidiano do trabalho em saude. Vitoria: EDUFES, 2001, p. 13-15.

MERHY, E. E. **Saude**: a cartografia do Trabalho vivo em ato. 2. ed. Sao Paulo: Hucitec, 2002.

MERHY, E. E.; FRANCO, T. B. Productive Restructuring and Technological Transition in Health. In: **O processo de trabalho e a mudança do modelo tecnoassistencial na saude**. 1999. Dissertation (Master's Degree in Collective Health)- Postgraduate Program in Collective Health, Unicamp, Campinas, 1999.

Merhy, E.E.; Franco, T.B. Por uma Composigao Tecnica do Trabalho Centered on relational technologies. (www.professores.uff.br/tuliofranco).

MERHY, E.E.; ONOCKO, R. (org). **Acting in Health, a challenge for the public.** Sao Paulo: Hucitec, 1997.

MINAYO, M., C. de S. **O desafio do conhecimento**: pesquisa qualitativa em saude. 7.ed. Sao Paulo: Hucitec, 2000.

MINAYO, M., C. de S. Qualitative-Quantitative: opposition or complementarity. **Cadernos de Saude Publica**, Rio de Janeiro, v. 9, n. 3: 239-62, 1994.

MINAYO, M.C.S (org). **Pesquisa Social**: teoria, metodo e criatividade. 19 ed. Sao Paulo: Vozes, 2001.

MINAYO, Maria Cecilia de Souza. **The challenge of knowledge:** qualitative research in health, 1997.

NUNES, M. O.; TRAD, L. B.; ALMEIDA, B. A. The community health worker: constructing the identity of this hybrid and polyphonic character. **Cad. Saude Publica**. Rio de Janeiro, v.18, n. 6, nov./dec. 2002. Available at: <http://www.scielo.br//>. Accessed on: June 20, 2006.

OLIVEIRA, R. G.; NACHIF, M. C. A.; MATHEUS, M. L. O trabalho do agente de saúde na percepção da comunidade de Anastacio, Estado do Mato Grosso do Sul. **Maringa**, v. 25, n. 1, p. 95-101, 2003. Available at: <http://www.ppg. uem.br/>. Accessed on: June 20, 2006.

WORLD HEALTH ORGANIZATION. **Alma Ata 1978**: Primary health care. Report of the International Conference on Primary Health Care. Brazil. WHO, 1979.

PAIM, J S and ALMEIDA FILHO, N de. **The crisis of public health and the utopia of collective health**. Salvador: Casa da Qualidade, 2000.

PAIM, J.S. **Modelos Assistenciais**: reformulando o pensamento e incorporando a protecção e a promoga da saude. In: Paim, J.S. Saude - politica e reforma sanitaria. Salvador: Cooptec/ISC, 2002.

PEDUZZI, M. **Multiprofessional health team**: the interface between work and interaction. 1998, 254 f. Thesis (Doctorate) - Postgraduate Program in Collective Health,

Faculty of Medical Sciences, State University of Campinas, 1998.

POPE, C.; MAYS, N. **Qualitative research in health care**. 2 ed. Porto Alegre: Artmed, 2005.

RIBEIRO, E. M.; PIRES, D.; BLANK, V. L. Theorizing about the health work process as an instrument for analyzing work in the Family Health Program. **Cad. Saude Publica**, Rio de Janeiro, v.20, n. 2, mar. /abr. 2004. Available at: <http://www.scielo.br/ />. Accessed on: July 20, 2005.

ROLNIK, S. **Sentimental cartography**: contemporary transformations of desire. Rio Grande do Sul: Sulina, 2006.

ROZANI, T. M.; STRALEN, C. J. **Dificuldades de Implantação do Programa de Saude da Familia como Estrategia de Reforma do Sistema de Saude Brasileiro.** Available at: <http://www.nates.ufjf.br/novo/revista/v6n2.htm>. Accessed on: May 26, 2005.

SANTANA, M. L.; CARMAGNANI, M. I. Family Health Program in BRAZIL: a focus on its basic assumptions, operationalization and advantages. **Saude e Sociedade**, Rio de Janeiro, v. 10, n. 1, jan/jul. 2001. Available at: <http://apsp.org.br/saudesociedade.htm/>. Accessed on: August 15, 2005.

SANTOS, S. B.; BARROS, E. B. **Trabalhador da Saude**: Protagonismo dos Trabalhadores na Gestao do Trabalho em Saude. Rio Grande do Sul: Unijul, 2007.

SCHERER, M.D. A; MARINO, S. R. A.; RAMOS, F. R. S. Ruptures and resolutions in the health care model: reflections on the Family Health Strategy based on Kuhnian categories. **Revista Interface-Comunicação, Saude, Educagao**. Botucatu: 2005, v. 9, n. 16. Available at: <http: //www.scielo.br//>. Accessed on: May 2, 2006.

SCHIMITH, M. D.; LIMA, M. A. Acolhimento e vinculo em uma equipe do Programa

Saude da Familia. **Cad. Saude publica**. Rio de Janeiro: v. 20, n.6, nov/dez. 2004.

SILVA, J. A.; DALMASO, A. S. The community health agent and his attributions: the challenges for the processes of training human resources in health. **Interface-Communication, Health, Education**. Botucatu: v.6, n. 10, feb 2002. Available at: <http: //www.debates. br/>. Accessed on: June 10, 2006.

SILVA, J. A.; DALMASO, A. S. The community health agent and his attributions: the challenges for the processes of training human resources in health. **Interface-Comunicagao, Saude e Educagao**, v. 10, n. 6, 2002. Available at: <//www.debates.br/>. Accessed on: June 10, 2006.

SILVA, J. A.; DALMASO, A. S. W. **Agente comunitario de Saude**: o ser, o saber, o fazer. Rio de Janeiro: FIOCRUZ, 2006.

SILVA, M.J.; RODRIGUES, R.M. - The community health agent in the process of municipalization of health. **Revista Eletronica de Enfermagem**. Goiania: v.2, n.1, jan/jun. 2000. Available at:< http: //www.fen.ufg.br/revista/>. Accessed on: July 10, 2005.

SILVA, M.R. F; JORGE, M.S.B. Professional practice in the PSF: representations and subjectivities. **Revista Brasileira de Enfermagem**. Brasilia: v. 55, n. 5, p. 549-555, 2002.

STARFIELD, Barbara. **Primary Care**: balancing health needs, services and technology. Ministry of Health. Brasilia: UNESCO, 2002.

Light Technologies and the Relational Field. **Saude em Debate**. Rio de Janeiro, v.27, n. 65, Sep/Dec 2003.

Light Technologies and the Relational Field. **Saude em Debate**. Rio de Janeiro, v.27, n. 65, Sept/Dec 2003.

TEIXEIRA, C. F. Health promotion and surveillance in the context of the regionalization of health care in the SUS. **Cad. Saude Publica**. Rio de Janeiro: v. 18, suppl., 2002. Available at: <http: //www.scielo.br//>. Accessed on: July 20, 2005.

TRIVINOS, A. N. S. **Introdupao a pesquisa em Ciencias Sociais**. Sao Paulo: Atlas, 1987.

VASCONCELOS, E. M. **The prioritization of the family in health policies**. Available at: <http://geocities.yahoo.com//>. Accessed on: 17 Feb. 2006.

VASCONCELOS, E. M. **Educapao popular e a atenpao a saude da familia**. Sao Paulo: Hucitec, 1999.

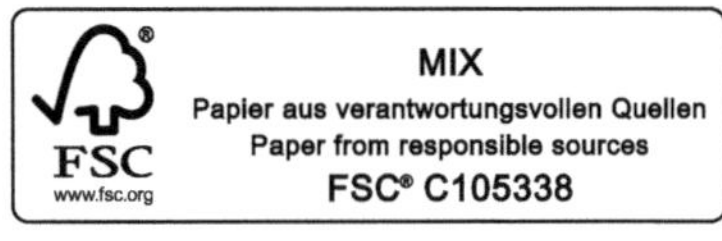

Printed by Books on Demand GmbH, Norderstedt / Germany